THE ULTIMATE PREGNANCY WORKOUT GUIDE

Nurturing the Health And Wellness Of Expectant Mothers

By

Joyce Allen

Table of Contents

CONCLUSION

INTRODUCTION

The Ultimate Pregnancy Workout Guide is a comprehensive resource designed to empower and support expectant mothers in maintaining a healthy and active lifestyle throughout their pregnancy. This guide emphasises the importance of exercise during pregnancy and provides valuable insights into creating a safe and effective workout plan.

The benefits of exercise during pregnancy are numerous and extend beyond physical fitness. Regular physical activity helps manage weight gain, improves circulation, boosts mood, reduces pregnancy discomforts, and enhances stamina. It also promotes better sleep, reduces the risk of gestational diabetes and preeclampsia, and aids in postpartum recovery. Engaging in exercise during pregnancy can also foster a sense of empowerment and self-confidence, enabling women to better cope with the challenges of pregnancy.

Addressing safety concerns is crucial when it comes to exercising during pregnancy. The guide emphasises the importance of consulting with a healthcare professional before starting any exercise program to ensure individual suitability and discuss any potential risks. Understanding the body's changing needs and limitations during pregnancy is key to designing a safe and effective workout routine. Certain exercises may need to be modified or avoided based on high-risk pregnancies or specific medical conditions.

Designing an effective workout plan for pregnancy requires consideration of the unique physiological and anatomical changes that occur. Low-impact activities such as walking, swimming, and prenatal yoga are generally safe and effective choices for most pregnant women. Strengthening exercises that target the core, pelvic floor, and major muscle groups help maintain stability, alleviate back pain, and prepare the body for the demands of pregnancy, labour, and postpartum recovery.

Listening to one's body is essential throughout the pregnancy journey. Expectant mothers should pay attention to how their bodies feel during and after exercise and make necessary adjustments. Avoiding exercises that cause pain, dizziness, or shortness of breath is crucial. Modifications and adaptations may be necessary as the pregnancy progresses. Staying flexible and modifying exercises to accommodate changing needs and limitations is important for ensuring a safe and comfortable workout routine.

The emotional and mental well-being of expectant mothers is also addressed in this guide. Pregnancy is not only a physical journey but also an emotional and mental one. Exercise has been shown to have a positive impact on mental health and overall well-being. Regular physical activity during pregnancy reduces stress, anxiety, and depression, enhances mood, and improves body image. Incorporating mindfulness techniques, deep breathing exercises, and relaxation practices into the workout routine further enhances the emotional benefits of exercise.

CHAPTER ONE

The Value Of Exercise During Pregnancy

During pregnancy, exercise has a considerable positive impact on both the mother and the foetus. The conventional wisdom that pregnant women should avoid exercise has been disproven by more recent research. Theoretically, women who exercised during pregnancy ran the danger of having smaller babies and of going into labour too soon. According to a recent meta-analysis involving more than 2000 women, aerobic exercise and moderate-intensity strength/toning exercise performed three or four days a week throughout the pregnancy were not linked to an increased risk for preterm births or infants with low birth weight. This was the case even for normal-weight women carrying singletons and having straightforward pregnancies. Only approximately 40% of patients exercise, despite doctors' advice to start or continue an exercise program throughout pregnancy. A pregnant patient can be easily inspired to make changes to both her and the unborn child's health. These suggestions must be applicable, though, and the doctor must follow up frequently. Exercise can relieve certain common aches and pains and even get the body ready for childbirth.

Deep vein thrombosis, a serious health concern that puts both the mother and the unborn child in danger, is linked to a sedentary lifestyle during pregnancy. Obesity can be caused by, or at least significantly contribute to, a sedentary lifestyle. In the United States, obesity is on the rise, and being obese while pregnant increases the chance of serious consequences. Obese patients are more likely to experience spontaneous abortions. Additionally, they are more likely to experience hydrocephalus, spina bifida, and other neural tube problems. The risk of gestational diabetes, preeclampsia, sleep apnea, macrosomia, preterm birth, and even stillbirth increases in obese pregnant patients. The chance of stillbirth increases with a woman's BMI. These women are safe to exercise, and it is recommended. Even patients who had previously been inactive are urged to begin an exercise regimen early in pregnancy. Additionally, it is regarded as safe in some high-risk pregnancies, including those with gestational diabetes and persistent hypertension. We'll talk about contraindications afterwards.

A woman's life is transformed and joyful throughout pregnancy. Numerous changes, both bodily and emotional, are brought about by it. Regular exercise is essential for keeping good health during pregnancy. Contrary to popular opinion, exercising during pregnancy can offer a number of advantages for both the mother and the unborn child. This goes against the notion that pregnancy should be a time of rest and inactivity. This essay discusses the value of exercising during pregnancy and focuses on how it improves overall pregnancy experience as well as physical and mental health.

Benefits to Physical Health: Pregnancy-related exercise has several positive effects on one's physical health. Pregnant women who regularly exercise can better their cardiovascular health, control weight gain, and lower their risk of gestational diabetes. It improves muscular strength and tone, which can help with labour and delivery. Exercise also encourages better posture, which helps ease pregnancy-related discomforts like back pain and pelvic girdle pain. Reducing the risk of issues like pre-eclampsia and gestational hypertension during pregnancy can also be accomplished by maintaining a healthy weight and enhancing cardiovascular health.

Psychological Health: Hormonal changes brought on by pregnancy can cause anxiety, melancholy, and mood swings. It has been demonstrated that regular exercise during pregnancy improves mental health. Exercise increases the production of endorphins, or "feel-good" hormones, which can help manage stress, elevate mood, and lessen depressive symptoms. Physical activity can help women adjust to their changing bodies and appreciate the beauty of pregnancy by boosting self-esteem and body image.

Reduction in the Risk of Pregnancy problems: Exercise has been linked to a decreased risk of some pregnancy problems. Regular exercisers have a lower risk of developing gestational diabetes, which can have both immediate and long-term health effects on both the mother and the unborn child. Exercise can also help prevent weight growth that is excessive, which lowers the risk of issues including macrosomia (a huge baby) and the requirement for delivery interventions. Exercise also helps to improve circulation, which reduces the chance of Deep Vein Thrombosis (DVT), a potentially fatal blood clot disorder.

Better Foetal Health: Regular exercise throughout pregnancy has a good impact on the developing baby's health. Exercise has been found in studies to boost blood flow to the placenta, giving the foetus a better supply of oxygen and nutrients. Improved delivery outcomes may result from healthier foetal development brought on by this increased blood supply. Exercise has also been linked to a reduced chance of preterm birth, which is a major worry for many pregnant moms. Babies that are delivered at full term often have a higher chance of developing and growing in a healthy way.

Guidelines for Exercise During Pregnancy: While exercise is safe for both the mother and the unborn child during pregnancy, there are a few rules that must be followed. Before beginning or continuing an exercise regimen during pregnancy, expectant moms should speak with their healthcare physician. Based on the woman's pre-pregnancy fitness level, any pre-existing medical conditions, and the stage of pregnancy, the intensity, duration, and type of exercise should be tailored to her needs. For the majority of pregnant women, low-impact exercises like walking, swimming, prenatal yoga, and stationary cycling are generally safe choices. It's important to pay attention to your body, drink plenty of water, wear supportive shoes, and stay away from activities that put you at risk for falls or impacts.

Function

Pregnancy-related conditions include macrosomia, gestational diabetes, preeclampsia, caesarean birth, low back pain, pelvic girdle discomfort, and urine incontinence have been proven to decline with exercise. Giving specific advice, such as which activity is safe and when she should start, is sometimes more effective when counselling a pregnant patient rather than just advising her that she should exercise. It is allowed for a patient to continue their usual exercise routine throughout pregnancy if they did so before becoming pregnant. If the activity involves a contact sport, it may be necessary to modify the intensity from time to time, or it may be safer to switch to a different activity altogether. The best exercise is thought to be aerobic. The heart pumps oxygenated blood to the working muscles during what is frequently referred to as cardiac activity. Large muscular groups (arms and legs) are repeatedly worked for an extended period of time. 150 minutes each week should be ideal. You can divide this up into shorter periods, like 30 minutes a day for five days a week. One can start an exercise regimen with as little as 5 minutes a day, and then gradually increase it by 5 to 10 minutes each week.

Walking, cycling, stair steppers, ellipticals, swimming, aerobic dancing, and yoga are typical forms of cardiovascular exercise. Exercise should be intense enough to raise the heart rate to between 110 and 120 beats per minute. (Although it varies with age, the typical pregnant woman is between the ages of 18 and 35.) The "talk test" is a useful tool for gauging workout intensity. A person is usually not overexerting if she can talk while exercising. Pregnancy issues might result from overexertion, thus it should be avoided. Walking is simple, cheap, and can be done both inside and outside. Pregnant women should pay strict attention to sufficient hydration and environmental temperature control, especially if they are just starting an exercise plan.

A mall, indoor track, or treadmill can offer a safe and protected setting for her to exercise in while pregnant in order to prevent overheating. Preventing dehydration and hyperthermia before and after exercise can be accomplished by drinking water. Since falling is more likely to happen when using a standard bike and could harm the pregnant patient and her foetus, cycling is best done on a stationary bike. Walking, which can strain the pelvic, may be less comfortable than cycling. Swimming is a great cardiovascular workout and is recommended if you have joint pain or other pregnancy-related discomforts. All the major muscle groups can be worked on in the weightless environment and buoyancy of the water. Excellent stretching and strengthening workouts that can also enhance mental well-being and lessen pain include yoga and pilates. These are only a few possible alternatives. Certain types of exercise should be avoided while pregnant. These include any contact sport (basketball, soccer, etc.), a sport that involves falling from a great height (skiing, skydiving, scuba diving), or one that involves high risk of injury (hockey, horseback riding).

Even if they have a history of engaging in strenuous exercise prior to pregnancy, women should keep an eye on themselves while exercising. During this phase, it's crucial to keep hydrated, reduce exposure to heat or humidity, and prevent hypoglycemia. Regular painful contractions, vaginal bleeding, dyspnea with effort, dizziness, headache, chest discomfort, or calf pain are all potential warning signs or symptoms. The pregnant patient should stop exercising and contact her doctor right once if these symptoms start to appear. Strenuous aerobic exercise and overexertion are not advised because they may divert blood flow from the foetal placental unit to the essential maternal organs, endangering the baby's health.

For the same reasons, heavy lifting and distance running are not recommended. The supine position, which puts pressure on the vena cava and compromises blood return to the heart and potentially compromises blood flow to the foetus, should be avoided by the pregnant patient.

Exercise is absolutely prohibited in cases of placenta previa, an incompetent cervix, bleeding during the second or third trimester, premature membrane rupture, preterm labour, substantial heart or lung problems, preeclampsia, or severe anaemia. To reduce their risk of thromboembolism, doctors encourage patients with such high-risk illnesses to walk rather than exercise.

Clinical Relevance

To improve the outcome of their pregnancy and the health of the unborn child, women should start an exercise regimen. Although weight loss may happen as a result of a patient's change from a sedentary to an active lifestyle, it is not the intended outcome during pregnancy. It could have a negative effect. Prenatal exercise is important for weight loss after delivery.

Other Concerns

Most pregnancies are thought to be safe and good for exercise. It enhances both the mother's health and the baby's wellbeing. It is advised that women continue exercising after giving birth to reduce pregnancy weight gain and improve their general health. It's vital to remember that exercise of any kind is beneficial during pregnancy. Some ladies might choose to hire a personal trainer or join a gym. However, walking for 45 to 60 minutes each day is sufficient as exercise on its own. Another excellent workout that relieves pressure on the lower back is swimming. Exercise should not, however, be taken too far; excessive physical activity is not advised as it can cause a fall and endanger the health. The quantity of activity that is tolerable will decrease as the pregnancy progresses, although walking should still be done. Wear compression stockings when exercising to prevent leg edema. Regular exercise has benefits that go far beyond pregnancy; it can help you manage stress, enjoy the outdoors, reduce weight, lower your blood pressure and cholesterol, and, most significantly, boost your self-confidence.

Improving Healthcare Team Results
There is a lot of evidence that shows physical and emotional benefits of exercise for healthy pregnant women. Almost any sort of exercise can be done by a pregnant woman as long as there are no negative effects during the pregnancy. Of course, this calls for using common sense and steering clear of activities that could cause falls. Prenatal nurses or primary care doctors often monitor pregnant women, so they are in a perfect position to inform the patient about the advantages of exercise. Additionally, the pharmacist ought to take

advantage of the chance to inform expectant women who visit a retail pharmacy. As long as there are no negative side effects, the pregnant woman can continue exercising. The pregnant woman should be instructed to use compression stockings frequently and to relax with her legs raised, at the end of the day.

Pregnancy exercise has many advantages for both the mother and the unborn child. It supports greater physical health, including enhanced muscular tone, cardiovascular fitness, and weight management. Additionally beneficial to mental health, exercise lowers stress, elevates mood, and increases self-esteem. thus minimising the possibility of difficulties.

Understanding the benefits of exercise for you and your baby

Even when you are not a pregnant woman, it can be difficult to maintain a regular fitness routine. But studies have shown that being active while pregnant is not only safe, but it can also have some significant advantages for both the mother and the unborn child.

Benefits of Exercise During Pregnancy

• Weight gain is reduced. According to one study, mothers who exercised two to three hours each week throughout their pregnancies were 40% less likely than mothers who did not. Gaining less weight may not only make it simpler to return to your pre-pregnancy shape after giving birth, but it may also reduce your risk of having gestational diabetes, which is high blood sugar during pregnancy. Uncontrolled blood sugar levels might increase your risk of having a larger-than-average baby, which can make labour challenging.

• Prepare yourself better for labour and delivery.Giving birth is a difficult undertaking, but if you approach it with stronger muscles, improved breathing control, and enhanced endurance, it will go more smoothly than one of your toughest workouts to date. Additionally, you could require less medical assistance during labour and stay in the hospital for a shorter period of time.

• Improve your mental wellness.Exercisers, compared to sedentary moms-to-be, may have a better body image, more self-esteem, and more vitality. Additionally, they may be less likely to experience postpartum depression.

• Experience less back pain.A recent study found that nearly 70% of pregnant women suffered from back pain. However, strengthening the muscles in your back, glutes, and thighs can improve your posture and perhaps ease back pain.

Benefits of Exercise During Pregnancy for Your Baby

• Your infant receives a significant brain boost.Babies whose mothers exercised throughout pregnancy showed enhanced neurodevelopment and had brains that were more active and mature.

• He has a lower chance of being underweight.Regular exercise during pregnancy may prevent hypertension, which affects 6 to 8% of expectant mothers in the US. High blood pressure reduces the blood flow to the placenta, making it more difficult for your baby to get the oxygen and nutrition he needs and may result in low birth weight.

• He might have a stronger heart.Recent research suggests that babies of mothers who exercise may have hearts that are stronger and healthier. Researchers discovered that pregnant women who were physically active during their pregnancies had babies with lower heart rates both in utero and after birth, indicating that a mother's fitness was helping to make her baby's heart more fit.

• Your baby arrives more easily.According to studies, pregnant women who work out during their pregnancies are likely to have babies that exhibit fewer signs of foetal distress when they give birth.

Safe Ways to Benefit from Exercise
Pregnant women are advised to engage in physical activity for at least 30 minutes on most days of the week.

• Once you've discussed becoming active with your doctor, begin gradually. For novices, five minutes of daily walking is excellent as they progressively increase to the suggested half-hour.

• When you're ready, you can safely engage in sports like swimming, stationary riding, and even strength training with moderate weights.

• If you exercised before becoming pregnant, you can probably keep working out at the same level; just make sure to consult your doctor first.

• Always pay attention to your body's signals; if something doesn't feel right, stop exercising and see a doctor.

Exercise is essential for maintaining a healthy lifestyle, and pregnancy is a key time to start. Regular physical activity is advantageous for both the mother and the developing child. It also benefits the mother. In this part, we will examine the different advantages of exercise for pregnant women and their unborn children.

1.   Improved Maternal Health: Pregnancy exercise has a strong positive impact on maternal health. Regular exercise promotes a healthy heart and effective blood circulation by strengthening the cardiovascular system. Improved cardiovascular health lowers the risk of preeclampsia and gestational hypertension,

hich can be dangerous for both the mother and the unborn child.

2. Better Weight Management: Pregnancy frequently results in weight increase, and it's important to maintain a healthy weight for both the mother and the unborn child. By burning calories, boosting metabolism, and improving overall body composition, exercise helps to control weight gain. Regular exercise can also reduce weight gain that is too much, which lowers the chance of issues like gestational diabetes and caesarean birth.

3. More Energy: Exercise has been demonstrated to alleviate the symptoms of exhaustion and low energy that might accompany pregnancy. Exercises with a moderate level of intensity, like prenatal yoga or walking, can increase energy and lessen fatigue. Regular exercise also improves mood and lessens depressive and anxious symptoms, supporting general wellbeing throughout pregnancy.

4.   Better   Musculoskeletal   Health: The musculoskeletal system needs support as the body changes significantly throughout pregnancy. Exercise can help. Strengthening exercises, like swimming or pregnant Pilates, can aid with posture, flexibility, and muscle strength. This can make the mother's pregnant journey more comfortable by easing everyday aches and pains like back pain and joint stiffness.

5. Lower Risk of Gestational Diabetes: Pregnant women who have gestational diabetes experience elevated blood sugar levels. By increasing insulin sensitivity, regular exercise has been found to lower the chance of developing gestational diabetes. Exercise improves the body's utilisation of glucose, which controls blood sugar levels and lowers the risk of gestational diabetes.

. Improved Foetal Development: Pregnancy ercise has a good effect on the growing foetus. ording to research, frequent physical activity helps babies' brains develop and enhances their general cognitive ability. Exercise also encourages normal foetal growth and lessens the chance of issues like intrauterine growth restriction. Exercise increases blood flow, which helps the baby receive vital nutrients and oxygen for healthy development.

7. Better Labor and Delivery Results: Keeping active during pregnancy can help the labour and delivery process go more smoothly. The muscles needed for labour are strengthened by regular exercise, which increases their effectiveness and shortens the time it takes to give birth. Exercise also encourages increased endurance, which can help manage labour pain and reduce the need for interventions like epidurals or caesarean sections.

8. Faster Postpartum Recovery: Exercise helps the mother after giving birth as well as throughout pregnancy. Preparing the body for childbirth by leading an active lifestyle during pregnancy also speeds up the process of getting

back to your pre-pregnancy fitness levels. Regular exercise helps to maintain muscle mass, tone the body, and encourage healthy weight loss, which improves mood and general well-being.

9. Positive Mental Health: Exercise can play a crucial part in developing positive mental health. Pregnancy can be an emotionally taxing time. Endorphins, hormones that improve mood, are released when you exercise, which helps to lower tension, anxiety, and depressive symptoms. Prenatal exercise classes or other group activities can offer social support and a sense of community as well, which is good for the mother's mental health.

The Impact of Exercise on Pregnancy Discomforts and Common Conditions

Although being pregnant is a wonderful and life-changing experience for women, it can also result in a number of discomforts and health issues that may compromise the general wellbeing of expectant mothers. Fortunately, it has been demonstrated that regular exercise during pregnancy has many advantages, including easing discomforts and lowering the risk of common disorders. This chapter examines how exercise affects common diseases and pregnancy discomforts, offering insights into how physical activity might improve pregnant women' general health and wellbeing.

1. Exercise and Morning Sickness/Nausea: Common pregnancy discomforts include nausea and morning sickness. Exercise can actually help with these symptoms, despite the fact that it may

seem paradoxical. Walking or swimming are examples of light to moderate aerobic exercises that can increase blood circulation, lessen tension, and produce endorphins, all of which help to lessen nausea and morning sickness.

2. Exercise and Back Pain: Because of the strain on the spine and the extra weight, back pain is a common complaint during pregnancy. Exercises that support the back and ease discomfort include low-impact aerobics and prenatal yoga. These activities work the core muscles. Exercises that encourage flexibility and good posture might also help to reduce back discomfort.

3. Exercise and Gestational Diabetes: Pregnancy-related gestational diabetes is characterised by elevated blood sugar levels. Gestational diabetes can be managed and prevented with regular exercise. Exercise enhances insulin sensitivity, prevents weight gain, and controls blood sugar levels. It has been demonstrated that women who exercise at a

moderate level, such as brisk walking or swimming, have a lower risk of acquiring gestational diabetes.

4. Exercise and Edema: Edema, or swelling, is a frequent ailment throughout pregnancy, especially in the legs and ankles. By enhancing blood flow and reducing fluid retention, exercise can minimise edema. By keeping the muscles active and encouraging healthy fluid flow throughout the body, low-impact exercises like stationary cycling, swimming, or prenatal yoga can help to reduce edema.

5. Exercise and Constipation: Due to hormonal changes and pressure on the digestive system, constipation is another ailment that many pregnant women endure. Constipation can be eased with regular exercise and a diet high in fibre. Constipation is less common since exercise encourages improved digestion and stimulates bowel movements.

6. Exercise and Fatigue: During pregnancy, fatigue is a common symptom that is frequently related to hormonal changes and the body's increased physical needs. Regular exercise helps reduce weariness by boosting energy levels, enhancing mood, and strengthening cardiovascular health. Exercises with little impact, like walking or prenatal yoga, can provide you a much-needed energy boost and enhance the quality of your sleep.

7. Exercise and Preterm delivery: Expectant mothers are very concerned about preterm delivery, which is defined as giving birth before 37 weeks of gestation. Numerous studies indicate that regular exercise can lower the risk of premature birth during pregnancy. Exercise at a moderate intensity has been linked to enhanced foetal development, lower inflammation, and improved uterine function, all of which lessen the risk of preterm birth.

Beyond preserving physical fitness, exercise during pregnancy has several positive effects. It has a big effect on how uncomfortable and common ailments are for expectant mothers. Regular physical activity is essential for improving general wellbeing throughout pregnancy, from easing morning sickness to lowering the chance of preterm birth. To guarantee the safety and appropriateness for specific circumstances, a healthcare practitioner must be consulted before beginning or changing an exercise regimen. Expectant moms can improve their health, ease discomforts, and facilitate a healthy pregnancy journey by including exercise into their daily routine.

Boosting Mental And Emotional Well-Being Through Exercise

One of the best ways to beat the blues, feel energised, and release stress is through regular physical activity. A simple 30-minute workout elevates your happiness and quality of life regardless of your level of fitness or competence. A regular workout break is even more important for your physical and emotional health while pregnant. Pregnancy is emotionally challenging, especially after receiving an infertility diagnosis. You may feel happy and excited about being a parent one minute and worried the next. It's challenging to ride the emotional rollercoaster, so you need strategies for controlling those strong emotions. You can better handle the mental and physical difficulties that come with pregnancy by exercising.

In the first trimester, emotional stress is brought on by a hormone surge and a dread of miscarriage. Your energy levels increase as the hormone levels balance out in the second trimester, and you stop feeling as emotionally volatile. Exercise throughout the second trimester keeps your weight and general health stable and gets you ready for the big event. Your degree of anxiety usually increases again throughout the third trimester since you are probably worried about giving birth and the wellbeing of your unborn child. By this time, you probably feel very worn out because of the added weight and the baby's movement, which makes it hard for you to sleep. Even a little exercise throughout the third trimester is beneficial.

How Workouts Help

Exercise has a very positive impact on your mental health whether or not you are pregnant. Numerous studies have shown that exercise helps to preserve emotional health, but you probably already knew that. The "runner's high" is a real phenomenon. The benefits of exercise for mental health are listed below.

Exercise Has a Positive Effect on Depression and Anxiety: It is scientifically proven that exercise has a beneficial effect on depression and anxiety. Endorphins, the hormone that makes you feel good, are released more frequently when you exercise. And you don't need to complete a marathon to benefit from them. Anxiety and depression symptoms can be reduced with three to five 30-minute sessions of moderate, doctor-approved exercise each week.

According to the American Psychological Association, experts concur that exercise is exactly as effective as antidepressants in alleviating chronic mood disorders. According to one hypothesis, engaging in regular exercise causes your body to release serotonin and dopamine, two potent mood-enhancing chemicals that help you feel happier, calmer, more focused, and emotionally stable.

Exercise Reduces Stress: You can counteract the negative effects of stress on your brain by raising your heart rate, provided your doctor gives the go-ahead. Neurohormones like norepinephrine are stimulated to be released by the body when blood flow is increased. You'll experience better mood, reduced brain fog (also known as "Pregnancy Brain"), and better cognition. Additionally, you'll notice improved communication between your body's sympathetic and central nervous systems, which supports an ongoing balanced stress response. We are all aware of how harmful stress is to general health.

Exercise Encourages Better Sleep: You usually have no trouble falling asleep throughout your first trimester, but occasionally anxiety may keep you from getting a good night's sleep. You could have a hard time relaxing as your pregnancy progresses and the baby kicks and jabs harder. Your ability to sleep becomes extremely valuable once the baby is born.

Unbelievably, the ability of the body (and mind) to relax before bed is one of the long-lasting consequences of regular exercise. Regular exercise also helps your body's circadian rhythm, which tells you when it's time to start drifting off to sleep. Both doctors and sleep specialists concur that you shouldn't exercise too close to bedtime.

Exercise has exponentially positive effects on your mental health throughout pregnancy. In addition to feeling better physically, you are also enhancing your long-term physical health. Chronic diseases including diabetes, high blood pressure, and heart disease can be warded off with regular exercise. Additionally, the effects of exercise on anxiety and sadness may prevent postpartum depression or at least minimise its effects. If you have any worries about any mental or emotional problems you may be experiencing, always talk to your doctor.

The best exercise for you throughout your pregnancy will be decided by you and your doctor. Extreme sports will obviously have to wait till after the baby is born, but depending on your level of fitness before being pregnant, activities like lifting weights or running might be okay.

Exercises of a moderate intensity are typically suggested for elevating mood and maximising the advantages to mental health. If you're not used to regular exercise, start with 10-minute intervals three times per day until your stamina improves. For your mental health and the social side, which also helps to promote mental health, look for pregnancy fitness classes.

CHAPTER TWO

Safety First: Guidelines And Precautions

Exercise will reduce your risks of having a miscarriage (when a baby dies in the womb before 20 weeks of pregnancy), a premature baby (born before 37 weeks of pregnancy), or a baby born with low birthweight (less than 5 pounds, 8 ounces). if you and your pregnancy are healthy.

How much exercise do you need while pregnant?

A healthy pregnant woman needs at least 212 hours of moderate-intensity aerobic activity every week. Aerobic exercises cause your heart to beat faster and your breathing to become more rapid and deep. Moderate-intensity indicates you're active enough to sweat and raise your heart rate. A quick stroll is an example of moderate-intensity aerobic activity. If you can't converse normally throughout an activity, you're probably working too hard.

You do not have to complete all 212 hours at once. Instead, spread it out over the week. Do 30 minutes of exercise every day, for example. If this seems like a lot, divide the 30 minutes by doing something physical for 10 minutes three times per day.

Why is exercise important during pregnancy? Regular exercise can help pregnant women who are in good health:

• Maintain good mental and physical health. Physical activity can improve your mood and provide you with extra energy. It also strengthens your heart, lungs, and blood vessels and helps you stay fit.

• Relieve some of the most typical pregnancy discomforts, such as constipation, back pain, and swelling in your legs, ankles, and feet.

• Assist you in better managing stress and sleeping. Worry, tension, or pressure that you feel in response to events in your life is referred to as stress.

• Assist in lowering the risk of pregnancy issues such as gestational diabetes and preeclampsia. Gestational diabetes is a type of diabetes that can occur during pregnancy. It occurs when your body has an excessive amount of sugar (called glucose) in the blood. Preeclampsia is a type of high blood pressure that some women have after the 20th week of pregnancy or after giving birth. These disorders can raise your chances of having difficulties during pregnancy, such as premature birth (born before 37 weeks of pregnancy).

• Lower your chances of having a caesarean delivery (commonly known as a c-section). Caesarean birth is a surgical procedure in which your baby is born through a cut made in your belly and uterus by your obstetrician.

• Prepare your body for labour and birth. Prenatal yoga and Pilates can help you practise breathing, meditation, and other relaxing strategies that may help you manage labour pain. Regular exercise can help give you the energy and power you need to get through labour.

What sorts of activities are safe during pregnancy?

It is typically OK to continue your activities during pregnancy if you were healthy and active before getting pregnant. Consult with your Healthcare provider to be certain. If you play tennis, run, or engage in other strenuous activities, you might be able to carry on doing so while pregnant. Later in your pregnancy, as your belly grows bigger, you might need to change your activities or cut back on your workouts. Choose activities that you enjoy if your provider thinks it's okay for you to exercise. If you didn't exercise before becoming pregnant, now is a fantastic time to start. Talk to your provider about safe activities. Begin softly and gradually increase your fitness. Start with 5 minutes of action per day and gradually increase to 30 minutes per day.

These activities are normally safe during pregnancy:

• Going for a walk. A fast walk is an excellent workout that is gentle on your joints and muscles.

• Water exercises such as swimming. Your growing baby is supported by the water, and exerting yourself against it keeps your heart rate elevated. Additionally, it's kind to your muscles and joints. If you get low back pain while you do other workouts, try swimming.

• Riding an exercise bike. This is more secure than using a regular bicycle when expecting. You are less likely to tumble off a stationary bike than you are on a regular cycle even as your belly grows.

• Pilates and yoga classes. Alert your yoga or Pilates instructor to your impending pregnancy. After the first trimester, the teacher can help you adapt or avoid positions like lying flat on your back or on your stomach that may be dangerous for pregnant women.Prenatal yoga and Pilates programs are offered by a few gyms and community centres only to expectant women.

• Classes in low-impact aerobicsYou always have one foot on the ground or equipment during low-impact aerobics.Low-impact aerobics exercises include walking, riding a stationary bike, and using an elliptical machine. Low-impact aerobics put less strain on your body than high-impact aerobics. Both feet leave the ground at the same time during high-impact aerobics. Some examples are running, jumping rope, and jumping jacks. Inform your instructor that you are expecting so that they may help you modify your training as needed.

• Strength training.Strength exercise can help you gain muscle and strengthen your bones. Weight training is safe as long as the weights are not too heavy. Inquire with your service provider about your lifting capacity.

You don't have to be a member of a gym or own special equipment to be active. You can stroll in a safe environment or do fitness DVDs at home. Find methods to be active in your daily life, such as doing yard work or using the stairs instead of the elevator.

Limitations and Contradictions: Ensuring Safe and Effective Exercise

Physical activity during pregnancy provides various advantages for both the mother and the developing child. Exercise on a regular basis can help manage weight gain, relieve discomfort, improve mood, increase energy levels, and enhance general well-being. However, in order to maintain the safety and health of both the mother and the baby, it is critical to be aware of the limitations and contradictions connected with pregnancy workouts. This chapter highlights important concerns and guidelines for safe and effective pregnant exercise.

1. Individual Differences:
Pregnancy is an individual experience for each woman, with varying physical capacities, health issues, and medical histories. As a result, before beginning or continuing a fitness regimen during pregnancy, it is critical to consult with a

healthcare expert. Individual situations can be addressed by an obstetrician, midwife, or trained prenatal fitness professional.

2. Dangerous Activities:
Certain activities are more dangerous during pregnancy and should be avoided in general. Sports involving contact, such as soccer or basketball, increase the risk of stomach damage. Activities with a high risk of falling, such as horseback riding or skiing, can endanger the mother and baby's safety. Due to the hazards of decompression sickness and foetal oxygenation, scuba diving should be avoided. Furthermore, sleeping flat on your back for extended periods of time after the first trimester may constrict major blood vessels, thereby limiting blood flow to the baby.

3. Changes and alterations:
The body changes significantly as pregnancy advances, affecting exercise capacities. Weight increase, hormonal changes, changes in balance and stability, and a shifting centre of gravity

necessitate training modifications and adaptations. Exercises that entail jumping or abrupt changes in direction, for example, should be avoided due to increased joint laxity and the danger of falling. A maternity support belt, for example, can give comfort and stability for the developing belly. Gentle strength training and prenatal yoga, for example, can help improve posture and stability throughout pregnancy.

4. Paying Attention to the Body:

During pregnancy, women must listen to their bodies and pay attention to any signals of discomfort, pain, dizziness, shortness of breath, or other undesirable symptoms while exercising. Workout intensity and duration may need to be altered as the pregnancy advances. Pregnancy fatigue is frequent, and it is critical to emphasise rest and recuperation to avoid overexertion. Rather than straining the limits, exercise should attempt to maintain or enhance fitness levels.

6. Temperature Control:

Pregnant women are more heat sensitive and have a decreased ability to remove heat from the body. As a result, excessive heat exercises, such as hot yoga or strong outdoor workouts in hot and humid circumstances, should be avoided. Overheating can cause dehydration, disorientation, and even consequences such as heat exhaustion or heat stroke. To avoid overheating, it is critical to stay hydrated and exercise in well-ventilated environments.

When approached with caution and awareness of the restrictions and contradictions, exercise during pregnancy can be safe and beneficial. Consultation with a healthcare practitioner, listening to the body, and avoiding high-risk behaviours are all good places to start.

Precautions to Take to Ensure a Risk-Free Pregnancy Workout

Exercise during pregnancy is usually seen as safe and beneficial to both the mother and the baby. To ensure a risk-free pregnancy workout, it is critical to emphasise safety and take particular precautions. Expectant moms can maintain their fitness, lessen pregnancy pain, and promote general well-being by following these tips. This post will go over the most important safety precautions for a safe and efficient pregnancy workout regimen.

1. Consult with your healthcare provider: It is critical to consult with your healthcare physician or obstetrician before commencing any fitness program during pregnancy. They can give you tailored recommendations based on your medical history, current health status, and the special needs of your pregnancy.

2. Begin gently and listen to your body: If you were not previously active, it is critical to begin cautiously and gradually increase the intensity and duration of your workouts. Pay attention to your body's cues and reduce or discontinue any activity that produces pain, discomfort, or extreme weariness. Because pregnancy hormones might damage your ligaments, avoid overstretching and unexpected movements that can strain your joints.

3. Select low-impact exercises: Low-impact workouts are generally suggested during pregnancy since they lessen joint stress and the chance of injury. Walking, swimming, prenatal yoga, stationary cycling, or low-impact aerobics are all good options. These exercises deliver cardiovascular advantages without putting your body under undue strain.

4. Avoid high-risk activities: Certain activities represent a higher risk during pregnancy and should be avoided to safeguard the safety of both

the mother and the foetus. Contact sports, activities with a high risk of falling (such as skiing or horseback riding), hot yoga or hot Pilates, scuba diving, and workouts that require resting flat on your back after the first trimester are all examples.

5. Adjust exercises to your growing body: Your body changes dramatically as your pregnancy advances. Adapt your exercises to accommodate your expanding tummy and shifting centre of gravity. Choose wider stances, supportive footwear, good posture, and prevent rapid movements or jerks, for example. To avoid pressure on your abdomen, modify exercises that need you to lie flat on your stomach.

6. Stay hydrated and avoid overheating: To stay hydrated, drink lots of water before, during, and after your workouts. Avoid exercising in hot and humid weather since it can cause overheating and dehydration, both of which can be dangerous during pregnancy. Wear light, breezy

clothing and take regular breaks to cool down if necessary.

7. Wear appropriate clothing and equipment: Invest in supportive, well-fitting athletic shoes that give stability and cushioning to preserve your joints. Wear a supportive bra with adequate breast support to avoid discomfort and damage. Dress comfortably in moisture-wicking clothes that allows for unfettered mobility and aids in body temperature regulation.

8. Do pelvic floor exercises: The pelvic floor muscles support the expanding uterus and can become weaker during pregnancy. Regular pelvic floor exercises, often known as Kegel exercises, aid in the maintenance of muscle tone, the prevention of urine incontinence, and the promotion of postpartum recovery. For advice on proper technique and frequency, consult a healthcare expert.

9. Maintain proper posture and body alignment: Maintaining good posture becomes increasingly

crucial as your pregnancy continues. Avoid slouching by standing tall with your shoulders back and relaxed. When exercising, keep good body alignment in mind and avoid moves that strain your back or pelvic. To help maintain proper alignment, consider employing supportive props such as stability balls or pregnancy-specific support belts.

10. Pay attention to your body and rest when necessary: Pregnancy is a time of physical and hormonal changes, and weariness is frequent. Listen to your body and give it enough rest and recuperation time in between workouts. If you are very weary or experiencing

If you have any of the following symptoms: dizziness, shortness of breath, vaginal bleeding, or contractions, stop exercising immediately and seek medical attention.

Staying active during pregnancy has various advantages, but safety should always come first. Expectant women can enjoy a risk-free training regimen that benefits their health and well-being throughout pregnancy by following these safety considerations. Remember to consult with your doctor, alter exercises as appropriate, and pay attention to your body's cues. You can maintain your fitness levels and have a good pregnant journey if you take sufficient care and attention.

CHAPTER THREE

Designing Your Pregnancy Workouts Routine

You'll never forget the exhilaration (or pure dread) you felt when you saw those two blue or pink lines appear. And now that you're pregnant, you may be thinking what has to change and what should be left alone.

What's the good news? Staying active is at the top of the list of things to do over the next nine months.

And whether you want to keep up your existing workout program or start something new, we've got you covered. Here's everything you need to know about remaining active during your pregnancy, from cardio and weight training to stretching and core routines.

The Advantages of Exercising While Pregnant

If you just exercise to squeeze into a smaller pair of jeans, you may need to change your outlook (and priorities) now that you're expecting.

Exercise during pregnancy, according to the American College of Obstetricians and Gynecologists (ACOG), can reduce the risk of:

• Premature birth

• Caesarean section

• Rapid weight gain

• Preeclampsia, gestational diabetes, or hypertensive conditions

• Smaller birth weight

It's also a great method to:

• Keep up your physical fitness

• Alleviate low back pain (hello, expanding stomach!)

• Control depression and anxiety symptoms

• Lessen tension

• Enhance postpartum healing

Some activities can be adopted in each trimester to help the body through its physical changes while preparing for a smoother return to exercise postpartum, according to Brooke Cates, prenatal and postpartum fitness expert and owner of Studio Bloom.
I encourage a shift in focus to core and pelvic floor awareness, which can assist you in

developing a deeper core-based connection before the major changes occur.

Exercise safety advice for pregnant women

When it comes to pregnancy exercises, I believe there aren't many that should be dropped from your present routine. While the majority of exercises can be continued throughout each trimester, modifying and scaling back where needed can help increase strength, stability, and physical adaptability as your body changes. With that in mind, the ACOG has provided some general safety precautions to consider when exercising during pregnancy.

• Consult your doctor if you are new to exercise or have any health conditions that may preclude you from exercising.

• Hydrate thoroughly before, during, and after activity.

• Put on supporting apparel, such as a sports bra or belly band.

• Avoid being hot, particularly during the first trimester.

• Avoid resting flat on your back for an extended period of time, especially during the third trimester.

• Stay away from contact sports and hot yoga.

Cardiovascular exercise during all three trimesters

Walking, swimming, jogging, and stationary cycling are popular cardiovascular exercises during all three trimesters. Unless your doctor has advised you otherwise, follow the U.S. Department of Health and Human Services Physical Activity Guidelines for Americans, which encourage at least 150 minutes of moderate-intensity aerobic activity per week.

If you're used to undertaking high-intensity workouts like running or have a high level of fitness, the ACOG says you can continue these activities throughout pregnancy — with your doctor's permission, of course.

Pregnancy Exercises for the First Trimester
The first three months of pregnancy can be an emotional roller coaster. From euphoria and pure excitement to concern, worry, and even terror when you realise you're in charge of feeding, growing, and keeping this small soon-to-be human safe and healthy.

You can continue with your regular workout program in the first trimester as long as you are not deemed a high-risk pregnancy. A well-rounded prenatal fitness plan should include at least 150 minutes of cardiovascular activity per week, as well as two to three days of strength training activities targeting the major muscle groups. It should also concentrate on particular activities that will ease your pregnancy and prepare you for labour and delivering. (It may appear distant, but it will arrive before you realise it!)

One important aspect to prepare for changes in posture is to practise body awareness. Doing an exercise like the pelvic curl is a great way to begin working on spinal mobility and strengthening the abdominal muscles that will support your belly as it grows.

Pelvic Curl

• Lie on your back with your feet flat on the ground, hip-width apart and your knees bent.

• Inhale deeply to prepare, and then exhale as you tuck your pelvis (sometimes referred to as your "hips") so that your spine is imprinted on the floor.

• Hold the tucked position while exhaling and rolling through the action to bring your spine out of the impression, one vertebra at a time.

• When you get to your shoulder blades, stop.

• Take a deep breath in at the peak of the action, then let it out as you fold your body back down, putting one vertebra at a time down onto the floor until you reach your starting position on the back of your pelvis (or your "hips," as many people will refer to them).

Do 12 to 15 repetitions. Bring both of your legs all the way together for an additional difficulty.

Pelvic Brace

As long as you don't experience pelvic floor symptoms like painful erections or urgent urination, continue doing this throughout your pregnancy.

• Lie on your back with your feet flat on the ground, hip-width apart and your knees bent.

• Put your low back and pelvis in a "neutral" position. You can do this by creating a tiny space in your lower back (your back shouldn't be shoved into the floor) and resting on the back of your pelvis.

• Take a breath in to get ready, then let it out to gently close the urethra, vagina, and anus openings during a Kegel contraction. Observe how your lower abdominal muscles want to cooperate as you perform this contraction.

• Using the Kegel, slightly contract the lower abs. Exhale, then repeat the contraction while relaxing your pelvic floor and abs.

• Once or twice a day, perform two sets of 8 to 15 repetitions of 3- to 5-second holds.

Kneeling Push-ups
This exercise combines strengthening of the upper body and core.

• Lie on your stomach with your knees kept behind your hips. Then, lift yourself up onto your hands and knees.

• Pull your abdominals in (the pelvic brace), and as you inhale, slowly descend your chest toward the floor.

• As you push back up, exhale.

• Begin with 6 to 10 repetitions and progressively increase to 20 to 24.

Squats

Additionally, the first trimester is the best time to start squats! You can also utilise the leg press machine if you have access to a gym. Squats, particularly bodyweight squats, are safe to perform throughout pregnancy.

Additionally, keeping your lower body muscles strong is a fantastic method to protect your back, allowing you to lift objects with your legs rather than your back. This is because squats develop all the muscles in your lower body, including the quadriceps, glutes, and hamstrings.

• Place yourself in front of a couch with your back to it. Start with your feet at around hip width apart. To guarantee appropriate form, use the couch as a reference.

• Squat as if you're about to sit on the couch, but stand back up as soon as your thighs make contact with the couch.

• Be sure to allow 5 seconds to descend and 3 seconds to ascend.

• As you squat, exhale; as you stand, inhale.

• Perform two 15–20 rep sets.

Related Article: 5 Safe Pregnancy Squat Techniques

Biceps Curls

This easy-yet-powerful manoeuvre is a favourite all during pregnancy. Bicep curls, according to

Jeffcoat, are a crucial exercise to incorporate into your exercises since you need to prepare your arms for frequently lifting and holding your infant.

• Holding 5- to 10-pound dumbbells, take a position with your knees slightly bent and your feet somewhat wider than your hips.

• As you slowly flex your elbows to bring the dumbbells up to your shoulders, exhale.

• After taking a breath, steadily reduce the weights again.

Lift the dumbbells for 3 seconds, then descend them for 5 seconds.

• Perform two sets of 10–15 reps each.

According to Brittany Robles, MD, CPT, some changes and additional strength training exercises to incorporate during the first trimester include:

• stepping lunges

• glute bridges (you can add ball squeezes in between your thighs during the glute bridges if you have a history of pelvic pain with pregnancies or are currently suffering any pelvic pain).

• Repetitive pushups
High-intensity interval training (HIIT) should be placed on hold during the first trimester of pregnancy, according to Robles, as it is a simple method to exhaust yourself at this point in the pregnancy.

Robles also advises staying away from any physical activity that puts you in danger of injury, such contact sports.

Pregnancy Exercises For the Second Trimester

Over the following few weeks, you might experience a sense of peace and even an increase in energy as the realisation that you're in this for the long haul settles in. This is the trimester when most women report feeling their best, so it's a great time to concentrate on your exercise regimen. However, I have highlighted the necessity for a little extra caution when engaging in strenuous activity due to the uterus's growing size.

I advise against engaging in any high-impact exercises that require jumping, sprinting, balance, or tiredness during the second trimester. Additionally, you should refrain from any workout that requires you to lie on your back for an extended amount of time. Consider adding some squat variations, such as single-leg squats, wide stance squats, and narrow squats, in addition to the workouts from the first trimester. Another exercise to incorporate during this trimester is the incline pushup, which works the shoulders, triceps, and chest.

The concept of strengthening the core as the abdomen expands is considerably simpler, now that the core foundation has been formed. And because things are starting to change and expand even more at this point, she frequently advises expectant mothers to keep working on stabilisation strength with a special emphasis on the inner thighs and glutes.

Incline Push-ups
• Stand with your back against a ledge or railing and spread your hands out on the ground shoulder-width apart.

• With your back straight, step your body back into a standing plank position.

• Slowly bring your chest down toward the railing or ledge while bending your arms.

• Straighten your arms to get back to your starting position.

• Perform two sets of 10–12 reps each.

Hip Flexor and Quadriceps Stretch

The second trimester is the best time to create a stretching practice that concentrates on the hip flexors, quadriceps, low back, gluteals, and calves because of postural changes.

The tummy tends to fall forward as a result of your shifting centre of gravity, shortening your hip flexor muscles. Stretching when pregnant can be done safely with this workout.

• Kneel down on the ground in a half-kneeling position. With your left foot in front of you and your left foot flat on the ground, place your right knee on the ground.

• Lunge toward your left foot while maintaining a tall posture until the front of your right hip and thigh feel stretched.

• Continue for a further two times after releasing after 30 seconds.

• Repeat while switching sides.

Side-lying Leg Lifts

Strengthening your balance and pelvic stabilising muscles is crucial to preparing for your shifting centre of gravity.

• Stack both of your bent legs on top of one another as you lay on your right side.

• Lift your right side off the ground just enough so that your waist is separated from the floor. Your pelvis will level as a result.

• Straighten your left leg and slant it forward slightly. Your toes should be pointing down toward the ground as you rotate your hip.

• Take a 3-second exhale as you elevate your leg; a 3-second inhale as you lower it. Make sure you maintain the small space you generated between your waist and the floor as you lift your leg.

Mermaid Stretch

Your diaphragm and ribs may begin to feel pressure as your baby grows, which could be uncomfortable.

• Lie on the ground with your feet facing to the right and your knees bent (or folded).

• As you inhale, raise your left arm straight up to the ceiling; as you exhale, side bend your torso to the right. In this instance, the left side should experience the stretch. Hold for four long, calm breaths. If you are having pain on your left side, you should stretch in this direction.

• If the right side bothers you, turn around. In the second trimester, begin stretching in both directions to lessen the likelihood of this happening.

Pregnancy Exercises For The Third Trimester

As your body starts to get ready for labour and delivery, you'll undoubtedly notice a slowdown during the third trimester, if not at times an abrupt halt. This is a wonderful time to concentrate on cardiovascular exercises, maintain your flexibility, and build your core strength with:

• Walking

• Swimming

• maternity yoga

• Pilates

• Pelvic Floor Exercises

• Bodyweight exercises

Your upper and lower body muscles will remain strong thanks to these.

Jeffcoat advises against engaging in any workout that increases your danger of falling, for your own safety. It's a good idea to stay away from exercises that could cause you to lose your balance, fall, or have an abdominal impact that could harm your unborn child because your centre of gravity is changing every day, she advises.

Pubic symphysis discomfort, which is pain in the front pubic bone, is another prevalent complaint. Jeffcoat advises staying away from exercises that require you to spread your legs too far because doing so will make the pain worse.

Diastasis Recti Correction
According to Jeffcoat, diastasis recti, or the separation of the rectus abdominal muscles, is a worry for women during this period. This condition manifests as a bulge that runs down the middle of your belly. She suggests

performing a diastasis recti corrective exercise to counteract this.

• Place a pillow beneath your head and shoulders while lying on your back. Feet are flat on the ground, and knees are bent.

• Lay a crib or twin sheet on your lower back (above your pelvis and below your ribs), rolling it so that it is about 3 to 4 inches wide.

• Take hold of the sheet and fold it once over your stomach. The sheet should then form an X as you pull each side as you hold the sides.

• Inhale deeply to become ready, then lift your head and shoulders off the pillow while pressing your back flat against the floor. You are softly "hugging" the sheet across your midsection during this move to assist your abs.

• Lower your breath in and out ten to twenty times. Start at 10 and work your way up if your neck or shoulders are sore.

• Repeat this twice daily.

During the third trimester, you should also focus on low-weight or bodyweight-only exercises for strength:

• Bodyweight squats or sumo squats performed with a wider stance for a larger base of support (if pelvic discomfort is not present)

• Light-weight standing shoulder presses

• Light weight bicep curls

• pressing up against a wall

• reshaped planks

• light-weight tricep kickbacks

The lesson

Being physically active during pregnancy is good for the mother and the unborn child.

Maintaining a strong core, toned muscles, and a healthy cardiovascular system can be accomplished by engaging in some type of exercise most days of the week. Additionally, it can improve your mental health tremendously (hurray for endorphins!).

Always pay attention to your body's cues and quit if you experience any pain or discomfort. As usual, if you have any queries or worries about how your body is adapting to a fitness regimen, speak with your doctor.

medical review completed on April 30, 2020

• Parenting

• Maternity

• Prenatal Care

Understanding the Different Components of Fitness During Pregnancy

Pregnancy is a transforming and one-of-a-kind time in a woman's life. It is a period in which the body goes through a slew of physiological and hormonal changes in order to accommodate the growth and development of a new life. Maintaining physical fitness at this time is critical for both the mother's health and the pregnancy's proper advancement. It is crucial to note, however, that the approach to exercise during pregnancy differs from ordinary workout programs. It necessitates a thorough understanding of the various components of fitness and how they are modified to meet the needs of a pregnant woman. In this chapter, we will look at different components of fitness and how they might be addressed when pregnant.

1. Cardiovascular Endurance: Cardiovascular endurance refers to the heart and lungs' ability to efficiently deliver oxygen-rich blood to working muscles.
The cardiovascular system undergoes considerable modifications during pregnancy. To support the growing foetus, the heart rate and blood volume rise. Maintaining cardiovascular fitness throughout pregnancy is critical for improving circulation, controlling weight gain, and lowering the risk of gestational diabetes and preeclampsia. Low-impact aerobic exercises like walking, swimming, stationary cycling, and prenatal aerobics programs are excellent for maintaining cardiovascular fitness without putting too much strain on the body.

2. Muscular Strength: Muscular strength refers to the muscles' ability to generate force. Certain muscle groups shift during pregnancy to support the developing abdomen and maintain

appropriate posture. During this time, the muscles of the pelvic floor, back, and abdominal region are especially crucial. These muscle group strengthening exercises can help relieve back discomfort, improve posture, and prepare the body for delivery. However, heavy lifting and activities that place undue strain on the abdominal muscles, such as traditional sit-ups, must be avoided. Under the supervision of a skilled instructor, prenatal yoga, Pilates, and resistance training with smaller weights or resistance bands can be useful.

3. Flexibility: The range of motion around a joint is referred to as flexibility. The body releases a hormone called relaxin as the pregnancy continues, which relaxes the ligaments and joints to accommodate the growing baby and prepare for birthing. While increased flexibility might be beneficial during labour, it can also cause joint instability and raise the risk of injury. Stretching exercises that target major muscle groups, such as the hips, back, and chest, can assist maintain flexibility while also preserving joint stability.

Prenatal yoga and moderate stretching practices are great options for increasing flexibility and promoting calm.

4. Balance and Coordination: Due to weight increase and changes in posture, pregnancy shifts the body's centre of gravity. This shift can have an impact on balance and coordination, increasing the likelihood of falls and accidents. Balance and coordination exercises can help pregnant women adjust to these changes and lessen the probability of an accident. Tai Chi, pregnant dance classes, and modified yoga poses that emphasise stability and body awareness can all be useful. It is critical to exercise with caution and avoid activities that pose a high risk of falling or collision.

5. Posture and Alignment: As the abdomen expands, so does the body's posture and alignment to accommodate the shifting weight. Backaches, neck pain, and discomfort can all be exacerbated by poor posture during pregnancy. It is critical to engage in exercises that strengthen

the back muscles and encourage proper posture. Prenatal Pilates, yoga, and activities that target the back and core muscles can assist to maintain appropriate posture and relieve discomfort.

6. Stress Management and Relaxation: Pregnancy can be a period of intense emotions, physical discomfort, and stress. It is critical to incorporate relaxation techniques and stress management measures into your fitness program for general well-being. Prenatal meditation, deep breathing techniques, and mild activities like prenatal yoga are all beneficial during pregnancy.
Massage and water treatment can help you relax and reduce tension. These activities can also aid in the improvement of sleep quality, which is frequently compromised during pregnancy.

It is important to remember that each pregnancy is unique, and that special considerations and adaptations may be required. Before beginning or changing an exercise routine during pregnancy, consult with a healthcare physician or a trained prenatal fitness instructor. They can offer tailored advice based on the individual's health, pregnancy progression, and any potential risks or issues.

Staying fit throughout pregnancy entails knowing and addressing the many components of fitness while taking into account the physiological changes and limits that occur with pregnancy. Pregnant women can improve their general well-being, manage discomfort, and prepare their bodies for the journey of birthing and parenting by integrating suitable exercises and adaptations.

Cardiovascular Exercises to Improve Endurance and Circulation

Staying active and maintaining cardiovascular fitness during pregnancy is critical for the mother's and developing baby's general health and well-being. Regular cardiovascular activity can assist improve endurance, circulation, weight management, minimise the risk of gestational diabetes and preeclampsia, and promote a healthy pregnancy. In this chapter, we will look at several safe and efficient cardiovascular exercises that can be added to pregnancy workouts to help with endurance and circulation.

1. Walking: Walking is a low-impact activity that is both safe and convenient for most pregnant women. It gives you a wonderful cardiovascular workout without placing too much strain on your joints. Walking on a daily basis can help you improve your endurance, strengthen your heart,

and increase your circulation. It is best to start slowly and progressively increase the time and intensity of the walks as tolerated. It is critical to invest in a decent pair of supportive and comfortable walking shoes to reduce any discomfort or foot-related disorders.

2. Swimming: Swimming and water aerobics are great cardiovascular exercises for pregnant women. The buoyancy of the water supports the weight of the growing abdomen, decreasing joint strain and allowing for fluid motions. Swimming works the entire body, including the arms, legs, and core muscles, and provides a good cardiovascular workout. It also aids in the relief of swelling and discomfort associated with pregnancy. Swimming or water aerobics for 30 minutes to an hour a few times a week will assist increase endurance, cardiac strength, and circulation.

3. Stationary Cycling: Using a stationary bike during pregnancy is a safe and effective cardiovascular exercise alternative. It is a

low-impact exercise that improves endurance and circulation while minimising joint stress. Stationary cycling also allows for easy resistance level modification, making it suited for people of varying fitness levels. To avoid lower back discomfort, it is critical to maintain appropriate posture and avoid excessive forward tilting. Cycling sessions that are gradually increased in duration and intensity can assist improve cardiovascular fitness over time.

4. Prenatal Aerobics: Prenatal aerobics programs tailored exclusively for pregnant women are an excellent technique to increase endurance and circulation. These classes often include low-impact movements accompanied by music, such as marching, stepping, and dancing. Prenatal aerobics programs are taught by certified instructors who understand the unique demands and limits of pregnant women. These programs offer a secure and supportive atmosphere in which individuals can engage in cardiovascular exercise while focusing on good form and making necessary adaptations.

5. Low-Impact Dance: Low-impact dance activities, such as Zumba or dance-based fitness courses designed specifically for pregnant women, can be a fun approach to improve cardiovascular health while pregnant. These programs use rhythmic movements and choreography to increase heart rate and circulation. It is critical to select programs created exclusively for pregnant women or to inform the instructor about the pregnancy to ensure that proper adaptations and safety precautions are implemented.

6. Elliptical Training: Using an elliptical machine during pregnancy can provide a low-impact cardiovascular workout. The elliptical action is easy on the joints while still giving a great cardiovascular and pulmonary training. Maintaining appropriate form, using the core muscles, and avoiding excessive tilting forward are also key. Gradually increasing the intensity and duration of elliptical exercises can

aid in the improvement of endurance and cardiovascular fitness.

7. Modified High-Impact workouts: Due to the increased pressure on the joints and the potential of falls or accidents, high-impact workouts such as jogging, jumping, or vigorous aerobic routines are generally not recommended during pregnancy. Some high-impact exercises, however, can be performed under the supervision of a healthcare physician or a skilled prenatal fitness instructor.

changed to be safer during pregnancy. Low-impact jumping jacks, for example, or modified running in place can provide a cardiovascular workout while lowering impact and stress on the body.

Considerations for Safety:
It is critical to prioritise safety and listen to your body when engaging in cardiovascular exercises during pregnancy. Here are some general safety precautions to remember:

1. Stay hydrated: To avoid dehydration, drink lots of water before, during, and after workouts.

2. Dress comfortably: Wear loose-fitting, breathable clothes that allow for flexibility of movement.

3. Wear the right shoes: Invest in supportive, comfortable shoes that give stability and cushioning.

4. Warm-up and cool-down: Always start your workouts with a modest warm-up to prepare your body and end with a cool-down to gradually lower your heart rate.

5. Avoid overheating: Exercise in a well-ventilated place, wear light clothing, and avoid hot and humid settings to avoid overheating.

6. Pay attention to your body: Be aware of any indicators of discomfort, pain, dizziness, or

shortness of breath. If anything doesn't feel right, it's critical to stop and seek medical attention if necessary.

Including cardiovascular activities during pregnancy workouts can help with endurance, circulation, and overall cardiovascular fitness. Pregnant women can maintain their fitness levels and reap the benefits of regular cardiovascular exercise by choosing safe and low-impact exercises such as walking, swimming, stationary cycling, prenatal aerobics, low-impact dance, elliptical training, and modified high-impact exercises. Remember to check with your doctor before beginning or changing any fitness plan during pregnancy to ensure it is safe and appropriate for your specific needs.

Exercises to Strengthen Key Muscle Groups

Strengthening activities are essential for maintaining general health and well-being when pregnant. They aid in the strengthening and support of the body as it transforms to accommodate the growing baby. Pregnant women can improve their posture, reduce discomfort, increase stability, and prepare their bodies for the physical demands of childbirth by targeting important muscle groups. In this chapter, we will look at some safe and efficient pregnant workout strengthening exercises for various muscle groups.

1. Pelvic Floor Muscles: The pelvic floor muscles are essential for supporting the pelvic organs as well as maintaining bladder and bowel control. These muscles are subjected to

increased tension and strain during pregnancy. Pelvic floor muscle strengthening can assist reduce urine incontinence and offer support for the expanding uterus. Kegel exercises are the most popular and effective method of targeting the pelvic floor muscles. To do Kegels, just contract and hold the muscles used to stop the flow of pee. Hold the contraction for a few seconds before releasing it. Throughout the day, try to complete several sets of Kegels.

2. Back Muscles: The back muscles, which include the erector spinae and the latissimus dorsi, are essential for optimal posture and spine stability. Back pain and stiffness are normal throughout pregnancy as the weight of the developing abdomen increases. Back muscular strengthening can help ease these symptoms. Among the most effective exercises are:

- Cat-Camel Stretch: Begin on your hands and knees, hands directly under your shoulders and knees directly under your hips. Arch your back toward the ceiling like a cat, then drop your back and raise your chest like a camel, bringing your shoulder blades together. Rep this movement, switching between cat and camel poses.

on your hands and knees with the Bird Dog. Extend your right arm forward while keeping your left leg straight back. Maintain a straight back and engage your core. Hold for a few seconds before switching sides and repeating.

- Resistance Band Rows: Attach a resistance band at waist height to a stable object. Hold the band's ends in both hands, palms facing each other. To produce tension in the band, take a step back. Begin by extending your arms in front of you, then push your shoulder blades together as you pull the band toward your chest. Release slowly and repeat.

3. Abdominal Muscles: It is critical to strengthen the abdominal muscles during pregnancy in order to support the expanding uterus, maintain proper posture, and prevent diastasis recti (abdominal muscle separation). However, it is

critical to select safe activities and avoid classic sit-ups or crunches, which can strain the abdominal muscles. Some safe and efficient abdominal exercises for pregnant women include:

- Pelvic Tilt: Lie on your back, legs bent, feet flat on the floor. Tilt your pelvis upward gradually, pressing your lower back into the floor. Hold for a few seconds before releasing. Repeat as needed.

- Standing or Sitting Side Bends: Position your feet shoulder-width apart while standing or sitting tall. Slowly slant your body to the side, placing one hand on your hip and elevating the other. Leaning forward or backward should be avoided, so keep your core tight. Do the opposite side and then revert to the starting position.

- Modified Plank: Begin by kneeling and placing your hands on the floor shoulder-width apart. Step your hands forward while extending your back legs. Keep your body in a straight line from head to toe. Hold for a few while before reducing gradually. You can modify this exercise as your pregnancy progresses by doing it against a wall or with the aid of a stability ball.

4. Gluteus maximus

Hips: During pregnancy, the glutes and hips are vital for stability, balance, and pelvic support. Strengthening these muscle groups can help relieve hip discomfort and keep the body stable as it ages. Among the most effective exercises are:

- Squats: Place your feet slightly wider than hip-width apart on the floor. Reduce your body weight to your heels as if you were sitting back in a chair. Lower your thighs until they are parallel to the floor, then push back up through your heels to return to the beginning position. Squats can be done with your body weight or with a stability ball against a wall for support.

- Clamshells: Lie on your side, bent knees piled on top of each other. Lift your top knee while maintaining your feet in contact with each other, keeping your feet together. Lower yourself back down and repeat. Repeat on the other side.

- Lie on your back, bend your knees, and place your feet flat on the ground to perform hip bridges. Form a straight line from your knees to your shoulders by pushing through your heels to lift your hips off the ground. Squeeze your glutes at the top, then slowly lower yourself back down.

5. Strengthening the chest and shoulder muscles will help with posture, counteract changes in the upper body, and lessen rounded shoulders. This is especially important during pregnancy. Specific muscle groups can be safely targeted by a few exercises:

Holding a pair of light dumbbells or resistance bands in each hand, sit on a stability ball or a chair with a backrest. Start by bending your arms 90 degrees so that your elbows are at shoulder level. The weights or bands should be advanced until your arms are fully stretched but not locked. Slowly re-enter the starting position and then repeat.

- Shoulder Rows: Holding light dumbbells or resistance bands in each hand, stand with your feet shoulder-width apart and your palms facing each other. Bring your hands to your shoulders by bending your elbows, then raise your arms back to their starting positions. Keep your shoulders relaxed and refrain from shrugging.

- Wall Push-Ups: Face a wall, arms extended, hands flat against the wall at shoulder height. Bend your elbows slowly, bringing your chest to the wall, and then push back to the beginning position. Adjust the distance from the wall as needed to enhance or lessen the difficulty. It is important to remember that each pregnancy is unique, and that particular considerations and adaptations may be required. Before beginning or changing an exercise plan during pregnancy, it is best to check with a healthcare physician or a competent prenatal fitness instructor. They can give you tailored advice based on your health, the stage of your pregnancy, and any potential risks or issues.

Finally, including essential muscle group strengthening exercises during pregnant workouts is critical for maintaining strength, stability, and general fitness. Pregnant women can support their changing bodies, alleviate discomfort, and prepare for childbirth by targeting the pelvic floor muscles, back muscles, abdominal muscles, glutes and hips, and chest and shoulder muscles. Remember to listen to your body, make changes as needed, and seek professional advice to maintain a safe and successful fitness plan throughout your pregnancy.

Flexibility and stretching routines for relaxation and improved posture

Stretching and flexibility exercises are essential components of pregnant training. They not only encourage relaxation and muscular relaxation, but they also help to improve posture, relieve discomfort, and prepare the body for the physical demands of labour. In this article, we will look at several safe and effective flexibility and stretching practices that can be added into pregnancy workouts to help with relaxation and posture.

1. Warm-up: It is critical to warm up the body before beginning any flexibility or stretching routine. A warm-up improves blood flow to the muscles, prepares them for stretching, and lowers the chance of injury. For a few minutes, a simple warm-up can involve easy motions like marching in place, arm swings, or modest

cardiovascular workouts like walking or stationary cycling.

2. Neck and Shoulder Stretches: Because of changes in posture and hormonal swings, the neck and shoulders frequently carry strain and discomfort throughout pregnancy. Stretching these areas can aid in the relief of muscle tension and the promotion of relaxation. Among the effective neck and shoulder stretches are:

- Neck Rolls: Tilt your head gently to one side, bringing your ear near your shoulder. Roll your head slowly in a circular motion from one side to the other. Rep in the other direction.

- Shoulder Rolls: In a circular motion, roll your shoulders up towards your ears, then back and down. Rep in each direction many times.

3. Stretches for the Chest and Upper Body: Pregnancy can create stiffness in the chest and upper body, resulting in rounded shoulders and bad posture. Stretching these areas can help open

up the chest, improve posture, and alleviate pain. Stretches for the chest and upper body that are useful include:

- Chest Opener: Stand tall, feet hip-width apart. Squeeze your shoulder blades together as you clasp your hands behind your back. Lift your hands away from your body, allowing your chest to open. Hold the stretch for a few seconds before releasing it.

- Upper Back Stretch: Sit on a chair or stability ball with your feet flat on the floor and stretch your upper back. Clasp your hands in front of you, rounding your shoulders and pulling your hands away from your body. Hold the stretch for a few seconds before releasing it.

4. Hip and Pelvic Stretches: The hips and pelvic area alter significantly as the baby grows. Stretching these areas can help relieve pain, increase flexibility, and prepare the body for labour. Among the effective hip and pelvic stretches are:

- Hip Circles: Stand shoulder-width apart with your feet shoulder-width apart and your hands on your hips. Circumcircle your hips clockwise, then counterclockwise. Allow your hips to move freely with soft and controlled movements.

- Butterfly Stretch: Sit on the floor with your feet touching and your legs forming a diamond shape. Gently press your knees into the floor until you feel a stretch in your inner thighs. In order to deepen the stretch, lean a little forward. Hold for a short while before letting go.

5. Gentle Spine and Lower Back Stretches: During pregnancy, the spine and lower back can feel discomfort and stress. Gentle stretching exercises can help relieve these symptoms and increase flexibility. Stretches for the spine and lower back that are effective include:

- Cat-Camel Stretch: Begin on your hands and knees, hands directly under your shoulders and knees directly under your hips. Arch your back like a cat, then lower it and raise your chest like a camel. Rep this movement, switching between cat and camel poses.

- Child's Pose: Bend your knees and sit back on your heels. Lower your upper body forward, extending your arms in front of you, and resting your brow on the floor or a cushion. Maintain your buttocks

Maintain touch with your heels while relaxing into the stretch.

6. Full-Body Stretches: Including full-body stretches in your pregnant workouts will aid in general flexibility and relaxation. Full-body stretches that are effective include:

- Forward Bend Standing: Stand tall with your feet hip-width apart. Bend forward slowly from the hips, reaching your hands to the floor or resting them on your shins. Maintain a tiny bend in your knees and allow your upper body to hang, feeling a nice stretch in your hamstrings and lower back. Hold for a few seconds before gradually rising back up.

- Modified Pigeon Pose: Begin on all fours, hands directly beneath your shoulders and knees beneath your hips. Bring one knee up behind your wrist, allowing your lower leg to rest diagonally behind you. Straighten the other leg back. Lower your upper body slowly toward the floor, feeling a stretch in the bent leg's hip. Hold for a few seconds before switching sides and repeating.

When including flexibility and stretching exercises into pregnancy training, keep the following safety precautions in mind:

- Pay attention to your body: During stretches, pay notice to any discomfort or pain. Avoid overexertion and alter or skip any stretches that don't feel right.

- Breathe deeply: During stretches, take deep breaths to encourage relaxation and allow for deeper stretching.

- Avoid bouncing by performing static stretches that last 20-30 seconds without bouncing or jerking.

- Stay hydrated: To stay hydrated, drink plenty of water before, during, and after workouts.

- Consult your healthcare provider: Before beginning or adjusting any workout or stretching plan, consult with your healthcare practitioner if you have any concerns or medical issues.

Finally, including flexibility and stretching routines into pregnancy workouts can help with relaxation, posture improvement, and overall well-being. Pregnant women can relieve discomfort, reduce muscular tension, and enhance flexibility by focusing on important regions such as the neck and shoulders, chest and upper body, hips and pelvis, spine and lower back, and implementing full-body stretches. Remember to listen to your body, stretch with caution, and get medical attention if you have any concerns or specific conditions.

CHAPTER FOUR

Nutrition And Hydration For Prenatal Fitness

Proper diet and hydration become critical during this stage for the health and well-being of both the mother and the developing infant. Maintaining a healthy diet and proper hydration not only helps the foetus grow and develop, but it also helps the mother's health. In this post, we will look at the importance of nutrition and hydration throughout pregnancy and present helpful tips for eating well and staying hydrated.

The Importance of Nutrition During Pregnancy: Proper nutrition is essential for a healthy pregnancy and foetal development. A pregnant woman's caloric needs rise to sustain the baby's growth as well as the changes in the maternal body. Here are some crucial nutrients to focus on throughout pregnancy:

1. Folic Acid: Folic acid is required for the creation of the neural tube and aids in the prevention of neural tube defects in babies. Folic acid-rich foods include leafy green vegetables, fortified cereals, legumes, and citrus fruits.

2. Iron: Iron is required for the creation of haemoglobin, which transports oxygen to the baby and aids in the prevention of anaemia in the mother. Lean meats, beans, spinach, and iron-fortified cereals are examples of iron-rich foods.

3. Calcium: Calcium is necessary for the growth of the baby's bones and teeth. It is also beneficial to the mother's bone health. Calcium is abundant in dairy products, leafy green vegetables, tofu, and fortified plant-based milks.

4. Protein: Protein is necessary for tissue growth and repair in both the mother and the infant. Lean meats, poultry, fish, eggs, dairy products, legumes, and nuts are all high in protein.

5. Omega-3 Fatty Acids: Omega-3 fatty acids, particularly DHA (docosahexaenoic acid), are essential for the brain and visual development of a baby. Fish, such as salmon and sardines, as well as walnuts, flaxseeds, and chia seeds, are high in omega-3 fatty acids.

Pregnancy Hydration: Proper hydration is equally crucial during pregnancy. Water aids in the maintenance of bodily fluid balance, digestion, nutrition transfer, and body temperature regulation. It also aids in the prevention of common pregnancy discomforts including constipation and edema. Here are some recommendations for staying hydrated:

1. Drink enough water: Pregnant women should drink at least 8-10 cups (64-80 ounces) of water per day. However, the precise amount may differ

based on factors such as climate, level of physical activity, and individual demands.

2. Keep an eye on urine colour: Urine colour can be a good sign of hydration status. Urine should ideally be light yellow or clear. Dark urine may suggest dehydration and the need for more fluids.

3. Include hydrating meals: Consuming hydrating foods, in addition to water, can help with overall hydration. Water-rich foods and vegetables, such as watermelon, cucumbers, and citrus fruits, can be useful.

4. Avoid coffee and sugary drinks: While moderate caffeine consumption is generally safe during pregnancy, excessive consumption should be avoided. Sugary drinks should also be avoided because they supply empty calories with no nutritious benefit.

5. Be conscious of your hydration needs while exercising: Pregnant women who exercise

should be especially mindful of their hydration needs. Water should be consumed before, during, and after workouts to replace fluids lost through sweating.

It is important to maintain sufficient nutrition and hydration during pregnancy for the health and well-being of both the mother and the developing baby. A well-balanced diet rich in important nutrients like f

The combination of folic acid, iron, calcium, protein, and omega-3 fatty acids promotes optimum embryonic growth. Furthermore, remaining appropriately hydrated by ingesting an appropriate amount of water and hydrating foods is critical for maintaining general health and reducing pregnant discomforts. Consultation with a healthcare professional or a certified dietitian is recommended to develop a personalised nutrition and hydration plan that meets individual needs and guarantees a healthy and pleasant prenatal journey.

Understanding the importance of proper nutrition during pregnancy

What is nutrition, and why is it important during pregnancy?

Nutrition is the discipline of eating a nutritious, well-balanced diet to supply your body with the nutrients it needs. Nutrients are nutritional components that our bodies require in order to function and thrive. Some of them are carbohydrates, lipids, proteins, vitamins, minerals, and water. Nutrition is more crucial than ever when pregnant. Many critical nutrients are required in greater quantities than before pregnancy. Making good meal choices every day can help you provide your kid with the nutrients he or she requires to develop. It will also assist in ensuring that you and your baby grow the appropriate amount of weight.

Do I have any unique dietary requirements now that I'm pregnant?

More folic acid, iron, calcium, and vitamin D are required than before pregnancy:

• Folic acid is a B vitamin that may aid in the prevention of certain birth abnormalities. Pregnancy requires 400 mcg (micrograms) per day. During pregnancy and breastfeeding, you require 600 mcg per day from foods or supplements. This amount is difficult to obtain through diet alone, therefore you must take a folic acid supplement.

• Iron is essential for your baby's brain development and growth. Because the volume of blood in your body rises during pregnancy, you require more iron for yourself and your growing baby. Every day, you should consume 27 mg (milligrams) of iron.

• Taking calcium while pregnant helps lower your chance of preeclampsia, a dangerous medical disease that causes an abrupt rise in blood pressure. Calcium also strengthens your baby's bones and teeth.

• Pregnant women should consume 1,000 mg (milligrams) of calcium each day.

• Pregnant adolescents (ages 14-18) require 1,300 mg of calcium each day.

• Vitamin D aids calcium in the formation of the baby's bones and teeth. Every woman, pregnant or not, needs 600 IU (international units) of vitamin D each day.

It is important to remember that taking too much of a supplement might be dangerous. Extremely high doses of vitamin A, for example, can result in birth abnormalities. Take only the vitamins and minerals that your doctor has recommended. When pregnant, you also require more protein. Beans, peas, eggs, lean meats, shellfish, and unsalted nuts and seeds are all good sources of protein.

Another important nutritional concern during pregnancy is hydration. When pregnant, your body requires considerably more water to be hydrated and nurture the life within you. As a result, it's critical to drink plenty of fluids every day.

What should I expect to gain during my pregnancy?

How much weight you should acquire is determined on your health and your pre-pregnancy weight:

• If you were normal weight prior to pregnancy, you should gain 25 to 35 pounds.

• You should gain more weight if you were underweight before pregnancy.

• If you were overweight or obese prior to becoming pregnant, you should acquire less weight.

Consult your doctor to determine how much weight gain is safe for you during pregnancy. During your pregnancy, you should gain weight gradually, with the majority of your weight gained in the fourth trimester.

Do I need to consume extra calories while pregnant?

The number of calories you require is determined by your weight-gain objectives. Your health care provider can advise you on what your target should be based on factors such as your pre-pregnancy weight, age, and rate of weight gain. The following are general recommendations:

• You generally don't need any extra calories during the first trimester of pregnancy.

• During the second trimester, you typically require an additional 340 calories.

• During the third trimester, you may require an additional 450 calories per day.

• You may not require extra calories in the latter weeks of pregnancy.

It's important to remember that not all calories are the same. Consume nutritional foods rather than "empty calories" found in soft drinks, candies, and desserts.

Which foods should I avoid when pregnant?
You should avoid the following foods while pregnant:

• Alcoholic beverages.There is no known safe amount of alcohol for a pregnant woman to consume.

• Fish containing high levels of mercury.White (albacore) tuna should be limited to 6 ounces per week. Tilefish, shark, swordfish, and king mackerel should not be eaten.

• Foods more likely to contain bacteria that might cause foodborne disease, such as

• Smoked seafood that has been refrigerated, such as whitefish, salmon, and mackerel

• Unless blazing hot, hot dogs or deli meats

• Preserved meat spreads

• Salads from the store, such as chicken, egg, or tuna salad

• Soft unpasteurized cheeses such as feta, Brie, queso blanco, queso fresco, and blue cheeses

• Any type of raw sprout (including alfalfa, clover, radish, and mung bean)

Excessive caffeine consumption.Caffeine consumption in excess may be detrimental to your infant. Caffeine in little to moderate levels (less than 200 mg (milligrams) per day) appears to be safe during pregnancy. This is equivalent to around 12 ounces of coffee. However, more research is required. Check with your doctor to see if consuming a small amount of caffeine is safe for you.

Pregnancy Exercise Hydration Guidelines for Optimal Performance and Well-Being

It is important to stay hydrated for overall health and well-being, especially during pregnancy. Adequate hydration is even more important when exercising during this period. Pregnancy activities provide various advantages, including greater cardiovascular fitness, reduced pain, and improved mood. Pregnant women, on the other hand, must pay special attention to their hydration demands in order to maximise performance and protect the well-being of both themselves and their developing baby. In this post, we'll go over hydration guidelines for pregnant women who exercise, highlighting the necessity of water intake, indicators of dehydration, and tactics for staying hydrated.

The Importance of Pregnancy Hydration:
Water is required for a variety of physiological functions including as nutrient transport, temperature regulation, and waste elimination. Because of the increased blood volume and the additional demands placed on the body during pregnancy, sufficient hydration is even more important. Hydration is especially crucial during exercise because it helps regulate body temperature, prevents dehydration, and promotes organ and tissue health.

Pregnant Women's Hydration Recommendations:
1. Drink Plenty of Water: The most basic rule for staying hydrated during pregnant activities is to drink plenty of water. Pregnant women should strive for a total daily water intake of roughly 2.3 litres (about 10 cups), according to the American College of Obstetricians and Gynecologists (ACOG). This quantity, however, may differ depending on individual characteristics, exercise levels, and weather

conditions. Consult a healthcare professional to assess your individual hydration requirements.

2. Pre-Exercise Hydration: It is critical to begin exercising hydrated. To establish optimal hydration levels, drink 16-20 ounces of water 1-2 hours before exercising. Consider taking an additional 8-10 ounces of water just before beginning the workout session if it is longer or more strenuous.

3. Hydrate During Exercise: Pregnant women should drink fluids on a regular basis to replace fluids lost by sweating. During activity, aim to drink 7-10 ounces of water every 10-20 minutes. However, depending on factors such as intensity, duration, and individual sweat rates, this may vary. Monitoring your body's indications and thirst sensations can also help you determine your hydration requirements.

4. Electrolyte Balance: Because exercise can cause electrolyte imbalances, it's critical to replace these vital nutrients. Include

electrolyte-rich items in your diet, such as bananas, oranges, yoghurt, and leafy greens. Additionally, sports drinks or electrolyte-enhanced water can be used to restore electrolytes lost through sweating during extended or vigorous exercise sessions.

5. Post-Exercise Rehydration: It is critical to refill fluids after completing an exercise to restore hydration levels. Drink 16-24 ounces of water for each pound of body weight lost when exercising. Monitoring urine colour might be a useful tool for determining hydration status. Dark pee signifies dehydration, while pale yellow urine shows sufficient hydration.

Dehydration Warning Signs to Look Out For:
It is important to be aware of the indicators of dehydration during pregnancy activities. Some examples of common indicators are:

- Thirst
- Dry or sticky lips

- Fatigue or dizziness
- Low urine output or dark urine
- Headache
- Muscle cramps
- Rapid heartbeat

If you develop any of these symptoms, you must immediately cease exercising, rest, and rehydrate. Severe dehydration can be dangerous for both the mother and the baby, therefore it is best to seek medical assistance if symptoms persist or worsen. Hydration is essential for sustaining peak performance and well-being throughout pregnancy activities. Adequate water consumption is critical for sustaining physiological processes, maintaining body temperature, and ensuring overall health.

Pregnant women can engage in physical activity safely and optimise the advantages of exercise during this special time by following the hydration standards listed above and listening to their bodies' cues. Remember to contact a healthcare provider to evaluate your unique hydration requirements and make any required adjustments depending on personal circumstances and activity intensity. remain hydrated, remain active, and have a fit and healthy pregnancy.

CHAPTER FIVE

Postpartum Recovery And Returning To Exercise

Nurturing your body during postpartum period

Exercise after pregnancy might help you feel your best. Consider the benefits of fitness after pregnancy, as well as techniques to keep motivated.

One of the best things you can do for yourself after pregnancy is exercise. Take note of these recommendations to get started securely.

Regular exercise after pregnancy can:
• Help with weight loss, especially when paired with calorie restriction

• Increase your cardiovascular fitness.

• Tone and strengthen the abdominal muscles

• Boost your energy level

• Policy

• Chances

• Ad Options

Physical activity can also help:

• Relieve stress

• Encourage better sleeping habits

• Relieve postpartum depression symptoms

Better still, incorporating physical activity into your daily routine allows you to set a positive example for your child now and in the future.

Exercise and breastfeeding

Moderate exercise is not thought to affect breast milk quantity or quality, or your baby's growth. It's critical to stay hydrated while nursing. Keep a water bottle ready during your workout and drink lots of fluids throughout the day.

Some study suggests that high-intensity exercise may cause lactic acid to collect in breast milk, producing a sour taste that a baby may not like, but this is very unlikely.

Consider feeding your baby before working out or pumping before working out and feeding your baby the breast milk you just pumped afterward if intense exercise is a priority during the first few months of nursing. Alternately, work out first, take a shower, express a few millilitres of milk, and then offer the breast after 30 or 60 minutes.

When should you begin?

If you had an uneventful pregnancy and vaginal delivery, it's normally okay to start exercising a few days after giving birth or as soon as you feel ready. If you had a C-section, significant vaginal repair, or a complex birth, consult with your doctor about when to begin an exercise regimen.

<u>Objectives for physical activity</u>
After pregnancy, the Department of Health and Human Services recommends at least 150 minutes of moderate-intensity aerobic activity each week, preferably spaced out over the week, for most healthy women. Consider the following recommendations:

• Create time to warm up and cool down.

• Start slowly and gradually increase your speed.

• Stay hydrated.

• Wear a supportive bra and nursing pads if you're breastfeeding in case your breasts leak.

• Stop exercising if you get pain.

Activities to try

Begin with something low-impact and uncomplicated, such as a daily walk. If you want to meet other new moms, check for a postpartum exercise class at a nearby gym or community centre.

Consider the following exercises, with the approval of your doctor:

Pelvic tilt. Do the Pelvic tilt a couple times everyday to strengthen your abdominal muscles. Lie on your back with your knees bent on the floor. In order to flatten your back against the floor, contract your abdominal muscles and gently raise your pelvis. Hold for as long as ten seconds. Five times, then escalate to ten to twenty repetitions.

• The Kegel exercise. Strengthen the muscles that support the uterus, bladder, small intestine and rectum. Kegel exercises might reduce urine and anal incontinence when performed often. As if you were attempting to stop urinating in midstream, tighten the muscles in your pelvic floor. Between contractions, hold for up to 10 seconds before relaxing for the same amount of time. Per day, try to complete at least three sets of ten repetitions. Do not perform Kegel exercises while urinating.

• A happy baby yoga position. Your pelvic muscles may tense and feel unpleasant after giving delivery. You can relax and gently stretch your muscles with the use of this yoga position to lessen pain. Kneel down on the floor with your back to the wall. Widen your hips a little more than your knees. Grab onto the outside of your feet or ankles with your hands while maintaining your arms on the inner of your knees. In order to drop your knees to the ground, bend your knees so that the bottoms of your feet are facing upward. Then, gently lift your feet off the ground. Focus on relaxing your pelvic muscles as you attempt to hold this stance for 90 seconds.

What is postpartum care?

The postpartum phase is the first six weeks following childbirth. For mothers, this is a joyful moment, but it is also a period of adjustment and healing. You'll bond with your baby during this period, and you'll have a post-delivery visit with your doctor.

Getting Used to Being a Mother
It is tough to return to normal life after the birth of a child, especially if you are a new mother. While it is vital to look after your child, you must also look after yourself.

After giving delivery, the majority of new mothers do not return to work for at least six weeks. This allows you to adjust and establish a new normal. You may experience sleepless nights since a baby has to be fed and changed regularly. It can be both irritating and exhausting. The good news is that you'll ultimately settle into a routine. Meanwhile, here are some things you can do to make the transition easier:

1. Get enough rest.To deal with exhaustion and fatigue, get as much sleep as possible. Your infant may require feeding every two to three hours. Sleep when your baby sleeps to ensure adequate rest.

2. Look for help.Accept help from family and friends without reluctance throughout and after the postpartum period. Your body requires rest, and practical support around the house can assist you in getting it. Friends and family members can assist with meal preparation, errands, and child care in the home.

3. Eat healthful foods.Consume a nutritious diet to aid recuperation. Increase your intake of whole grains, vegetables, fruits, and protein. Drink plenty of fluids, especially if you're breastfeeding.

4. Exercise.Your doctor will tell you when it is safe to exercise. The workout should be easy for the body. Take a stroll across your

neighbourhood. A change of scenery is energising and might help you feel more energised.

Putting together a new family unit

A new baby is an adjustment for the entire family and may change the dynamic of your relationship with your partner. It is also possible that you and your partner will spend less quality time together during the postpartum period, which can be challenging. There are ways to manage throughout this difficult and stressful period.

Be patient at first. Recognize that every relationship undergoes changes with the birth of a kid. It will take some time to adjust, but you will do so. Caring for your newborn baby gets easier with each passing day.

Also, communicate as a family. If someone in the family, whether it's a spouse or other children, feels left out, talk about it and be understanding. Despite the fact that children require a lot of attention and that you and your partner will spend the most of the day caring for their needs, don't be afraid to spend time alone as a couple during the postpartum period.

Postpartum Depression and Baby Blues
The baby blues are very typical during the postpartum period. This is frequent within a few days of giving birth and can last up to two weeks. In most cases, you will not have symptoms all of the time, and they will vary. 70% to 80% of new mothers experience mood swings or negative sentiments after giving birth. Baby blues are caused by hormonal fluctuations, and symptoms may include:
• inexplicable tears

• irritation

• sleeplessness

• melancholy

• alterations in mood

• nervousness

<u>When should you go to the doctor?</u>
The baby blues are not the same as postpartum depression.When symptoms linger for more than two weeks, it is considered postpartum depression. Other symptoms include feelings of shame and worthlessness, as well as a loss of interest in daily tasks. Some mothers suffering from postpartum depression withdraw from their families, have no interest in their infant, and have suicidal thoughts.

Postpartum depression necessitates medical attention. Consult your doctor if you are depressed for more than two weeks after giving birth or if you have thoughts of harming your kid. Postpartum depression can strike at any moment after giving birth, even a year later.

Adapting to Physical Changes
Along with emotional changes, you will experience physical changes such as weight gain

after giving birth. Be patient because losing weight does not happen overnight. Once your doctor has cleared you to exercise, start with a few minutes of moderate activity every day and progressively increase the length and intensity of your workouts. Take a stroll, swim, or enrol in an aerobics class. Losing weight also entails eating nutritious, well-balanced meals rich in fruits, vegetables, and whole grains. Every new mother loses weight at a different rate, so don't compare your efforts to those of other new mothers. Breast-feeding accelerates your return to pre-pregnancy weight since it improves your daily calorie burn.

If you have any questions or concerns regarding your body's changes during the postpartum period, consult your doctor. Other physical changes include:

Engorgement of the breasts
Your breasts will begin to fill with milk a few days after birth. Although this is a normal procedure, the swelling (engorgement) can be

painful. Engorgement becomes better with time. Apply a warm or cold compress to your breasts to relieve soreness. Breast-feeding nipples normally go away as your body adjusts. To relieve cracking and soreness, apply nipple cream.

Constipation

Drink plenty of water and eat high-fibre foods to increase bowel motion. Inquire with your doctor about safe drugs. Fibre, as well as over-the-counter treatments and sitting in a sitz bath, can help relieve haemorrhoids. Drinking water can help with urination issues after childbirth. Kegel exercises can help you strengthen your pelvic muscles if you have incontinence.

Pelvic floor modifications

The perineum is the region between the rectum and the vagina. It grows and tears regularly during birth. This area may be sliced by a doctor on occasion to aid your labour. Doing Kegel exercises, wrapping cold packs in towels and relaxing on a pillow can all help this area recover after birth.

Sweating
Hormonal changes after having a baby may cause evening sweating. Remove the blankets off your bed to stay cool.

Uncomfortable uterine symptoms
Cramping can be caused by a shrinking uterus following birth. With time, the soreness fades. Inquire with your doctor about pain medicines that are safe.

Discharge from the cervix
Vaginal discharge is common two to four weeks after birth. This is how your body gets rid of the blood and tissue in your uterus. Keep using sanitary napkins until the discharge stops.
Tampons and douche should not be used until your four to six week postpartum appointment, or until your doctor permits it. Using these

products in the first few weeks after giving birth may raise your risk of uterine infection. Inform your doctor if your vaginal discharge stinks. You may experience crimson spotting for the first week after giving birth, but excessive bleeding is not to be expected. Contact your doctor if you are experiencing excessive vaginal bleeding, such as wetting one sanitary pad within two hours. Giving birth will alter your family unit and routine, but you will adjust. Any emotional and physical changes that occur after pregnancy will gradually improve. Talk to your doctor about any worries you have, whether they are connected to depression, your baby, or the healing process.

Gentle exercises to promote healing and regain strength

You could require more time to recuperate from childbirth than you think. This is particularly true if you underwent a C-section. You can, however, start pelvic floor and abdominal muscle training exercises as soon as you feel ready.

If you had an episiotomy (a perineum incision to expand the entrance during delivery) or tore your perineum during birth, pelvic floor exercises can help you recover faster. Consult your doctor, midwife, or physiotherapist for further information.

Gentle Stomach Exercise

During pregnancy, your abdominal muscles separate down the middle. Make sure your muscles have healed before performing any strenuous abdominal activities, such as abdominal crunches.

Meanwhile, toning your stomach can be accomplished by engaging in an exercise that develops the deepest muscle layer (transversus abdominis). You can practise this exercise laying down, sitting, standing, or on your hands and knees.

Follow your doctor's, midwife's, physiotherapist's, or exercise physiologist's instructions, but here are some general guidelines:

• Keep your lower back flat.

• Exhale and draw your belly button closer to your spine. Your lower back should not be flexed or moved.

• Hold this position while lightly breathing. Count from one to ten.

• Take a deep breath and repeat each set up to ten times.

• Do 10 sets as many times as you can in one day.

• You might conduct your pelvic floor exercises concurrently.

Stage two Tummy Exercise

Once the space in your abdominal muscles has closed, you can progress to more demanding tasks. Some general guidelines are as follows:

• Lie on your back, bend your legs and your feet flat on the floor. Put your hands on your thighs.

• Exhale and lift your head and shoulders off the floor, contracting your abdominal. Raise your hands to your knees. Lift only your shoulder blades off the ground.

• Maintain a steady head and shoulders. Hold the position for a few seconds, then slowly lower your shoulders and head to the floor.

• For one set, repeat up to ten times.

• Aim for three sets every session.

Lower abdominal muscle strengthening exercises

The lower abdominal muscles are found beneath the belly button. Guidelines for working these muscles gently include:

• Check to see if your abdominal muscles have healed. Only do the 'gentle tummy workout' option until the gap is closed.

• Lie on your back, legs bent, and feet flat on the floor.

• Tighten your abdominal muscles.

• Slide your feet away from you slowly, striving to straighten both legs. The goal is to straighten your legs without arching your back.

• If your back begins to arch, come to a complete stop and slide your feet back towards your bottom.

• Aim for a total of 10 repetitions per set.

• Aim for three sets every session.

• As your lower abdominal muscles strengthen, you'll be able to move your feet more apart.

Exercises for the pelvic floor
The pelvic floor muscles support the colon, bladder, uterus (womb), and vagina. They are firmly draped between the tailbone (coccyx) and the pubic bone. Childbirth can weaken these muscles, leading to problems like incontinence later in life. You must first focus your attention on these muscles in order to train them. To aid

with identification, these are the muscles that you clench to cease urinating (weeing). These exercises can be done lying down, sitting up, or standing up.

Relax your abdominal muscles as much as possible. Don't bury your face or hold your breath. Squeeze and tighten the muscles gradually until they are as tight as they can be. Release carefully and softly. Then, execute the following exercises:

• Squeeze slowly and hold for five to ten seconds. Slowly let go. Rep 10 times more.

• Squeeze quickly, brief, and forcefully. Rep 10 times more.

• Squeeze, then cough lightly or clear your throat. Rep three times more.

• Aim for at least five or six sets per day.

Types of Postnatal Exercise

Remember that your ligaments and joints will be loose for at least three months after giving birth, so avoid any high-impact workouts or sports that involve quick direction changes. Excessive stretching should also be avoided. Postnatal exercise suggestions include:

• Fast walking

• Watersports

• Aerobics in water

• Yoga

• Pilates exercises

• Aerobic workouts with low impact

• Weight training using light weights

• Biking.

Consult your doctor for more advice and precautions.

Aerobic exercise recommendations in general

Follow the advice of your doctor or midwife, but here are some general guidelines:

• Allow yourself enough time to heal, especially if you had a caesarean birth.

• Before beginning any postnatal fitness program, consult with your doctor or midwife; you may be recommended to wait or modify your workouts.

• If you are having difficulty with the skills required for the aforementioned exercises, please seek the advice of a physiotherapist, exercise physiologist, or other adequately qualified and certified fitness professional.

• Aim for a weekly weight loss of roughly half a kilogram.

• Wear a bra that is supportive.

• Avoid any activities that put strain on the weak pelvic floor and hip joints until strength and stability improve. Be cautious of activities that entail abrupt changes in direction (such as high-impact aerobics, jogging, and contact sports). This changes according to the type of pregnancy and delivery you had.

• Begin by exercising for about five to ten minutes at a time.

• Ultimately, your exercise sessions should last between 30 and 50 minutes.

• Hydrate thoroughly before, during, and after activity.

• Don't push yourself too hard; if you're out of breath, slow down.

Don't be disheartened if your progress is slow; it may take months to return to your pre-pregnancy form and weight.

Signs that you should slow down
Don't push yourself too much. If you exercise too hard, your body may send you warning signals, which may include:

• Increased tiredness

• Aches and pains in the muscles

• Changes in colour from lochia (postpartum vaginal flow) to pink or red

• Increased lochia flow

• Lochia resumes its flow after a brief halt.

CHAPTER SIX

Holistic Approach TO Pregnancy Fitness

Pregnancy is a physically and emotionally transforming experience for women. Expectant mothers must prioritise their health and well-being while their bodies undergo multiple changes to accommodate the growing baby within. A comprehensive approach to pregnant fitness can give a plethora of benefits, assisting women in navigating the challenges of pregnancy and preparing for childbirth. In this post, we will look at the importance of a holistic approach to fitness during pregnancy, as well as the numerous factors that contribute to a well-rounded and balanced prenatal exercise regimen.

Physical Health

Maintaining physical fitness during pregnancy is critical for the mother's and developing baby's health. Regular exercise can help with typical aches and pains like back pain, exhaustion, and swelling. It also promotes better sleep and boosts cardiovascular health. However, before beginning any new fitness regimen, it is critical to customise the workout routine to the changing needs of the body and to obtain medical counsel. Walking, swimming, and prenatal yoga are all low-impact exercises that are highly advised throughout pregnancy. These activities offer gentle yet effective workouts that improve strength, flexibility, and endurance. Prenatal yoga, for example, involves breathing methods and gentle stretches to help relieve tension, improve posture, and boost relaxation.

Strength training, in addition to low-impact workouts, can be advantageous during pregnancy. Strengthening the pelvic floor and core muscles supports the developing belly, improves posture, and aids in an easier delivery. A trained prenatal fitness instructor or a healthcare provider can assist in developing a safe and appropriate strength training program.

Hydration and nutrition

Nutrition is critical to maintaining a healthy pregnancy and supporting the baby's growth and development. Taking a holistic approach to pregnancy fitness entails paying particular attention to diet and maintaining enough nutrition. A healthy diet rich in fruits, vegetables, lean meats, whole grains, and healthy fats provides critical nutrients for both the mother and the infant. It is also critical to stay hydrated during pregnancy. Water helps to maintain amniotic fluid levels, assists digestion, reduces constipation, and regulates body temperature. Adequate hydration is critical during exercise to avoid overheating and dehydration.

Mind-Body Relationship

Pregnancy is a time of tremendous physical and emotional development. A holistic approach to exercise throughout pregnancy entails cultivating the mind-body connection. Meditation, deep breathing exercises, and mindfulness practices, for example, can help reduce stress and anxiety, enhance sleep quality, and boost general well-being.

Prenatal massage is another great method for improving the mind-body connection. It relieves muscle tension, increases circulation, and produces relaxation. Hiring a professional prenatal massage therapist guarantees that the massage is suited to the special needs and safety concerns of pregnancy.

Rest and Recuperation

In the middle of the joy and expectation of expecting a new child, pregnant moms must emphasise rest and healing. Adopting a holistic approach to pregnancy fitness entails appreciating the value of rest and relaxation. Pregnancy is frequently associated with bodily discomforts, exhaustion, and hormonal changes.

Getting enough rest allows the body to rejuvenate, maintains the immune system, and promotes optimal performance. Creating a peaceful bedtime routine and listening to the body's cues for rest are all important parts of rest and healing during pregnancy. Relaxing activities, such as taking warm baths, mild stretching, or reading a good book, can also contribute to a well-rounded approach to pregnant fitness.

Community Assistance and Education
A holistic approach to pregnancy includes, in addition to focusing on physical and emotional well-being. Fitness entails searching out community support and education. Prenatal exercise programs and support groups provide an opportunity for pregnant mothers to connect with other women who are going through similar situations. It fosters a sense of community by providing a forum for people to share expertise, seek assistance, and build friendships. Participating in childbirth education seminars or workshops provides women with important

information about labour, delivery, and postpartum care. Understanding the physiological changes that occur during labour and adopting coping strategies can help relieve anxiety and enable expectant women to make informed decisions.

Adopting a comprehensive approach to pregnant fitness is important for expectant moms' general well-being and the healthy development of their newborns. Women can start on their pregnant journey with confidence and grace by including physical activity, right nutrition, cultivating the mind-body connection, prioritising rest and recuperation, and seeking community support and knowledge. It's vital to remember that every pregnancy is different, and working with a healthcare expert throughout the process is essential to ensuring a safe and effective approach to holistic pregnant fitness.

Stress Management and Self-Care as a Holistic Approach to Pregnancy Fitness

Pregnancy is a life-changing experience that causes both physical and emotional changes. It is a time of joy and anticipation, but it can also be fraught with tension and anxiety. Adopting a comprehensive approach to pregnancy fitness entails addressing self-care and stress management in addition to physical well-being. In this post, we will look at the importance of self-care and stress management throughout pregnancy, as well as different ways for encouraging a holistic approach to pregnant fitness.

Understanding the Effects of Pregnancy Stress

Stress is ubiquitous in everyday life, but it can have a substantial influence on both the mother and the developing baby during pregnancy. Preterm birth, low birth weight, and developmental difficulties have all been linked to high levels of stress. It can also exacerbate maternal health issues including hypertension and postpartum depression.

Self-care and stress management skills are essential for maintaining a healthy and balanced mind and body throughout pregnancy. Reduced stress levels allow pregnant mothers to establish a loving atmosphere for their personal well-being while also promoting their baby's optimal growth and development.

Pregnancy Fitness Self-Care Practices
Self-care entails nurturing and caring for oneself on both a physical and emotional level. It is even more vital to engage in self-care techniques that promote general well-being during pregnancy. Some self-care behaviours that can be incorporated into a holistic pregnant fitness routine are as follows:

1. Prioritising Rest: Adequate rest and sleep are critical for maintaining energy levels and general

health. Create a pleasant sleep environment, develop a calming nighttime routine, and pay attention to your body's indications for rest.

2. Gentle Exercise: Low-impact exercises, such as pregnant yoga or swimming, improve not only physical health but also relaxation and stress reduction. Consult a trained pregnant fitness instructor to create an exercise routine that is specific to your needs.

3. Nutrition: Eating a well-balanced, nutrient-dense diet benefits both the mother's health and the development of the baby. Include fruits and vegetables, whole grains, lean proteins, and healthy fats in your meals. Also drink plenty of water to stay hydrated.

4. Pampering Activities: Do things that make you happy and relax. Relax with a prenatal massage, a warm bath with relaxing essential oils, or a good book or movie.

5. Mindfulness and Meditation: Using mindfulness and meditation practices to reduce stress and create calm can help. Spend some time each day focusing on your breath, observing your thoughts without judgement, and cultivating a happy mindset.

Pregnancy Fitness Stress Management Techniques

Stress management during pregnancy is critical for both the mother and the baby's health. Here are some stress-reduction techniques that can be included into a pregnant exercise routine:

1. Deep breathing exercises, such as diaphragmatic breathing, can stimulate the relaxation response in the body and reduce stress. Breathe deeply and gently, filling your belly with air and slowly exhaling.

2. Mind-Body Practices: Participate in mind-body exercises such as prenatal yoga or Tai Chi. These activities promote relaxation and

stress reduction by combining physical motions with breath awareness and mindfulness.

3. Support System: Create a network of family, friends, and healthcare providers that can provide guidance, understanding, and emotional support during your pregnancy journey. If necessary, attend support groups or seek counselling.

4. Time Management: To reduce unneeded stress, prioritise work and manage your time properly. When feasible, delegate responsibilities and practice saying no to obligations that may overwhelm you.

5. Positive Affirmations: Use positive self-talk and affirmations to combat negative ideas and boost self-esteem. Remember to remind yourself of your strength and capability to manage any problems that come your way.

Encouragement of self-care and stress management as part of a holistic approach to pregnancy fitness is critical for expectant women' well-being and the healthy development of their newborns. Women can establish a happy and supportive environment during their pregnancy journey by prioritising self-care habits, managing stress effectively, and seeking support when needed. Remember that each pregnancy is unique, and it is critical to seek tailored counsel and support from healthcare professionals throughout this transforming period. Accept self-care and stress management as vital components of your holistic approach to pregnant fitness for a healthier and more joyful pregnancy journey.

Nurturing the Mind-Body Connection During Pregnancy and Beyond

The mind and body are inextricably linked, and this connection is amplified during pregnancy, a transforming journey that includes physical, mental, and spiritual changes. Nurturing the mind-body connection throughout pregnancy and beyond is critical for both the expectant woman and the developing baby's general well-being. In this article, we will address the importance of the mind-body connection during pregnancy, as well as its advantages and practical tactics for building and maintaining this connection during this transforming period and beyond.

Understanding the Pregnancy Mind-Body Connection

The mind-body link refers to the reciprocal interaction that exists between our mental and emotional emotions and our bodily feelings and responses. During pregnancy, the mind and body work together to support the baby's growth and development. Hormonal variations, bodily adaptations, and emotional swings all contribute to the mind-body interplay.

The Advantages of Fostering the Mind-Body Connection During Pregnancy

Developing the mind-body connection when pregnant has various advantages for both the mother and the baby. These advantages include:

1. Less tension and Anxiety: Pregnancy can cause tension and anxiety. Cultivating the mind-body connection through various practices can aid in the reduction of negative emotions and provide a sense of calm and relaxation.

2. Improved Emotional Well-Being: Pregnancy can cause a wide range of feelings, from joy and enthusiasm to dread and anxiety. Women can develop emotional resilience and handle these

feelings more easily by strengthening the mind-body connection.

3. Physical Health Improvement: The mind-body link has a direct impact on physical health. The body can function efficiently when the mind is calm and balanced. This can result in better sleep, digestion, circulation, and general physical health.

4. Bonding with the Baby: Having a strong mind-body connection enables pregnant moms to have a strong link with their baby. It improves the mother's sense of connection and communication with her unborn child.

Practical Pregnancy Strategies for Nurturing the Mind-Body Connection

1. Mindfulness Meditation: Mindfulness meditation entails paying attention to the present moment while remaining nonjudgmental. This practice fosters a strong feeling of present and assists women in tuning into the physical sensations and emotions that come with

pregnancy. Expectant mothers can strengthen their mind-body connection by practising mindfulness on a daily basis.

2. Prenatal yoga incorporates gentle exercises, stretching, and breath awareness. It improves physical health, flexibility, and relaxation. Yoga fosters the mind-body connection by emphasising conscious breathing, awareness, and a profound attention on the sensations of the body.

3. Breathing Exercises: Deep breathing exercises can be done anywhere, at any time, and produce immediate calm. Women can activate the body's relaxation response, reduce tension, and improve the mind-body connection by purposefully slowing their breath, breathing deeply with the nose, and expelling thoroughly through the mouth.

4. Body Scan: A body scan is a mindfulness exercise that involves bringing attention to different parts of the body in a systematic

manner, observing sensations, and releasing tension. This technique assists women in connecting with their bodies, releasing physical discomfort, and fostering calm.

5. Creative Expression: Journaling, drawing, or painting can be great tools for fostering the mind-body connection. These activities allow women to communicate their feelings, emotions, and experiences, which promotes self-awareness and a stronger connection to their inner selves.

Positive Affirmations: These are utterances that represent positive attitudes and objectives. Affirmations about pregnancy, childbirth, and parenting, when repeated, can help women build a happy mindset and enhance their mind-body connection. Affirmations such as "I trust my body's capabilities" are examples, "I embrace the changes my body is going through" or "I have the ability to give birth" can be empowering and caring.

Beyond Pregnancy, Nurturing the Mind-Body Connection

The mind-body connection formed during pregnancy can be nourished and enhanced throughout the postpartum period and beyond. Here are some tips for keeping the mind-body connection strong:

1. Self-Care: Make self-care activities that benefit your emotional and physical well-being a priority. Take breaks, engage in things you enjoy, seek encouragement from loved ones, or practice mindfulness in regular duties.

2. Maintaining a Regular Mindfulness Practice: Maintain a regular mindfulness practice, even if it is only for a few minutes every day. Mindfulness can assist in navigating the challenges of parenthood, as well as reducing stress and promoting a balanced mind-body connection.

3. Movement and Exercise: Participate in postpartum exercises that enhance physical

well-being and reconnect you with your body. Walking, yoga, and postnatal fitness programs can all assist to reestablish the mind-body connection.

4. Seek emotional assistance from family, friends, or support organisations. Connecting with others who are going through similar circumstances can assist sustain mental well-being and develop a feeling of community.

5. Make Rest and Recovery a Priority: Adequate sleep is essential for postpartum recovery and sustaining a strong mind-body connection. Pay attention to your body's demands, take pauses when needed, and emphasise sleep and relaxation.

Nurturing the mind-body connection throughout pregnancy and beyond is vital for both the mother and the baby's holistic well-being. Women can experience lower stress, increased physical and mental health, and a closer bond with their newborns by intentionally nurturing this connection through mindfulness practices, movement, self-care, and emotional support. Remember that each woman's journey is unique, so listen to your body, seek advice from healthcare specialists, and tailor these tactics to your own needs. Accept the power of the mind-body link to improve your pregnancy experience and encourage long-term well-being during your parenthood journey and beyond.

CONCLUSION

Congratulations! You have reached the conclusion of your pregnancy fitness journey, and now it's time to reflect on the incredible progress you have made. Over the course of this guide, we have explored various aspects of maintaining a fit and healthy lifestyle during pregnancy. From the importance of exercise and nutrition to mental and emotional well-being, you have gained valuable insights and tools to support you on this beautiful and transformative journey.

Throughout your pregnancy, you have likely experienced numerous physical and emotional changes. It's important to acknowledge that every woman's pregnancy is unique, and what works for one may not work for another. However, the underlying principles of maintaining fitness during pregnancy remain consistent: listen to your body, consult with your healthcare provider, and make choices that align with your individual circumstances and preferences.

One of the key takeaways from this guide is the significance of regular exercise during pregnancy. Engaging in physical activity can provide numerous benefits, such as improved cardiovascular health, increased energy levels, enhanced mood, and better sleep. However, it's important to choose exercises that are safe and suitable for pregnancy. Low-impact activities like walking, swimming, and prenatal yoga are excellent choices for maintaining fitness while minimising the risk of injury. Remember to warm up, cool down, and stay hydrated during your workouts, and always prioritise safety over pushing yourself too hard.

Another crucial aspect of pregnancy fitness is proper nutrition. Your body requires additional nutrients during this time to support both your own health and the development of your growing baby. Concentrate on taking a balanced diet that includes a variety of fruits, vegetables, whole grains, lean proteins, and healthy fats. Stay hydrated by drinking plenty of water and limit your intake of processed foods, sugary snacks, and caffeine. Remember that weight gain is a normal part of pregnancy, and it's important to nourish your body without obsessing over the numbers on the scale.

In addition to physical health, we have also emphasised the importance of mental and emotional well-being during pregnancy. Pregnancy can be a time of joy and excitement, but it can also bring about feelings of anxiety, stress, and mood swings. It's important to prioritise self-care and find ways to manage these emotions. Practice relaxation techniques, such as deep breathing and meditation, to reduce stress and promote a sense of calm. Surround yourself with a supportive network of family and friends who can offer guidance and encouragement throughout your pregnancy journey.

Remember, it's perfectly normal to have days when you feel less motivated or energetic. Pregnancy is a unique time in your life, and it's essential to listen to your body and adjust your fitness routine as necessary. Be gentle with yourself and celebrate every small achievement along the way. Even a short walk or a few minutes of stretching can make a significant difference in your overall well-being.

As your pregnancy progresses, it's essential to maintain open communication with your healthcare provider. They will monitor your progress, provide guidance on exercise and nutrition, and address any concerns or complications that may arise. Your doctor or midwife is your best resource for personalised advice based on your specific needs and circumstances. Don't hesitate to reach out to them whenever you have questions or uncertainties.

Finally, as you embark on this new chapter of your life, remember that pregnancy is a temporary state. While fitness and health should remain a priority, it's important to be patient with yourself and allow for necessary adjustments as you transition into motherhood. The focus will shift from maintaining fitness during pregnancy to postpartum recovery and caring for your newborn. Embrace this new phase with an open heart and a flexible mindset, knowing that your body has undergone an incredible journey and will continue to adapt and change.

The pregnancy fitness guide has provided you with a comprehensive understanding of how to maintain a fit and healthy lifestyle during pregnancy. By incorporating regular exercise, nourishing your body with a balanced diet, prioritising mental and emotional well-being, and seeking guidance from your healthcare provider, you have laid a solid foundation for a healthy pregnancy and a positive postpartum experience. Cherish this transformative time, celebrate your accomplishments, and trust in the amazing capabilities of your body. Wishing you a joyful and healthy pregnancy journey!